THE NEW
CALISTHENICS
• FORMULA •

Revolutionary Workout Routines to Transform
Your Physique with Bodyweight Training |
Injury-Free Exercises to Build Functional Strength,
Mobility & Boost Endurance

MIKE GILDON

TABLE OF CONTENTS

INTRODUCTION

Imagine waking up each morning feeling stronger, more agile, and full of energy, ready to take on whatever the day throws at you. You don't need a gym membership or expensive equipment to achieve this—you only need your own body weight and a commitment to push your limits. That's where calisthenics comes in. This book is your guide to mastering the art of calisthenics, a powerful and transformative form of exercise that's been around for centuries but is now more relevant than ever. Whether you're a seasoned athlete or just starting on your fitness journey, calisthenics offers a way to build strength, endurance, and flexibility in the most natural and effective way possible.

You might be wondering, "Why calisthenics?" In a world full of shiny gym machines and complicated fitness gadgets, calisthenics stands out because it's simple, accessible, and incredibly effective. This book is designed especially for men who want to harness the full potential of their bodies, sculpt a lean and muscular physique, and achieve peak fitness without relying on a gym. Whether you're a busy professional, a stay-at-home dad, or someone who's always on the go, calisthenics fits into your life seamlessly. By the time you finish this book, you'll have all the knowledge and tools you need to incorporate calisthenics into your routine, transforming not just your body but your confidence and overall well-being.

WHAT IS CALISTHENICS?

CALISTHENICS IS A FORM OF EXERCISE THAT USES YOUR OWN BODY WEIGHT TO BUILD STRENGTH, FLEXIBILITY, AND ENDURANCE. UNLIKE TRADITIONAL WEIGHT TRAINING, WHICH OFTEN RELIES ON EXTERNAL WEIGHTS LIKE DUMBBELLS AND BARBELLS, CALISTHENICS FOCUSES ON MOVEMENTS THAT ENGAGE MULTIPLE MUSCLE GROUPS AT ONCE. THINK OF EXERCISES LIKE PUSH-UPS, PULL-UPS, SQUATS, AND PLANKS. THESE ARE ALL CLASSIC CALISTHENICS MOVES THAT HAVE STOOD THE TEST OF TIME BECAUSE THEY WORK.

At its core, calisthenics is about mastering control over your own body. It's not just about lifting heavy weights or looking good in the mirror—though those can be nice bonuses—but about developing functional strength that translates into better performance in everyday activities. When you practice calisthenics, you're not just working out; you're training your body to move more efficiently, to be more resilient, and to withstand the physical demands of life.

One of the greatest advantages of calisthenics is its versatility. You can perform these exercises anywhere—at home, in a park, or even in your office during a break. All you need is some space and your body. This makes calisthenics a highly adaptable and sustainable form of exercise, especially in today's fast-paced world, where finding time for the gym can be a challenge.

Moreover, calisthenics is scalable. Whether you're a beginner or an advanced athlete, there's always a way to modify the exercises to match your fitness level. For instance, if a standard push-up is too challenging, you can start with knee push-ups and gradually work your way up. On the other hand, if regular push-ups become too easy, you can advance to more complex variations like one-arm push-ups or clap push-ups. This adaptability makes calisthenics an excellent choice for anyone looking to build a solid foundation of strength and then continually challenge themselves as they progress.

THE HISTORY AND EVOLUTION OF CALISTHENICS

CALISTHENICS MIGHT SEEM LIKE A MODERN FITNESS TREND, BUT ITS ROOTS GO BACK THOUSANDS OF YEARS. THE WORD "CALISTHENICS" ITSELF COMES FROM THE GREEK WORDS "KALLOS," MEANING BEAUTY, AND "STHENOS," MEANING STRENGTH. THE ANCIENT GREEKS WERE AMONG THE FIRST TO PRACTICE CALISTHENICS, USING IT AS A WAY TO PREPARE THEIR BODIES FOR BATTLE. THE EMPHASIS WAS ON BUILDING FUNCTIONAL STRENGTH, AGILITY, AND ENDURANCE—QUALITIES THAT WERE ESSENTIAL FOR SOLDIERS.

Fast forward to the 19th century, and calisthenics became popularized in Europe and the United States as part of physical education programs. Schools incorporated calisthenics into their curricula, recognizing its benefits for overall health and fitness. It wasn't just about building muscle; it was about creating a well-rounded physical conditioning program that could be practiced by people of all ages and abilities.

In the 20th century, calisthenics took a bit of a backseat as weightlifting and bodybuilding gained popularity. The rise of gyms and fitness centers meant that more people were turning to machines and free weights to build muscle. However, calisthenics never disappeared entirely. Military training programs around the world continued to use calisthenics as a foundational part of their conditioning routines, emphasizing its effectiveness in building functional strength.

In recent years, calisthenics has experienced a resurgence, thanks in part to the rise of street workout culture and the growing popularity of functional fitness. People are rediscovering the benefits of bodyweight training, realizing that it offers a level of versatility, convenience, and efficiency that traditional gym workouts often lack. Today, calisthenics is practiced by millions of people around the world, from elite athletes to everyday fitness enthusiasts.

WHY CHOOSE CALISTHENICS OVER TRADITIONAL GYM WORKOUTS?

IF YOU'VE EVER FELT INTIMIDATED BY THE GYM, OVERWHELMED BY THE SHEER NUMBER OF MACHINES, OR FRUSTRATED BY THE LACK OF RESULTS DESPITE SPENDING HOURS LIFTING WEIGHTS, CALISTHENICS MIGHT BE THE SOLUTION YOU'VE BEEN LOOKING FOR. HERE'S WHY YOU SHOULD CONSIDER MAKING THE SWITCH FROM TRADITIONAL GYM WORKOUTS TO CALISTHENICS.

COST-EFFECTIVE AND ACCESSIBLE

One of the biggest advantages of calisthenics is that it's free. You don't need a gym membership, expensive equipment, or a personal trainer to get started. All you need is your body and a willingness to push yourself. This makes calisthenics accessible to everyone, regardless of their financial situation or where they live.

Consider the long-term savings. Gym memberships can cost hundreds or even thousands of dollars per year, and that's before you factor in the cost of transportation, workout clothes, and supplements. With calisthenics, you can get in shape without spending a dime. Whether you're in your living room, a hotel room, or a public park, you can perform a full-body workout that rivals anything you'd get in a gym.

FUNCTIONAL STRENGTH AND REAL-WORLD APPLICATIONS

Calisthenics isn't just about building muscle—it's about developing functional strength that you can use in your daily life. Unlike traditional weightlifting, which often isolates specific muscles, calisthenics exercises engage multiple muscle groups simultaneously, mimicking the way your body naturally moves. This makes you stronger in a more holistic way, improving your ability to perform everyday tasks with ease.

For example, a standard gym workout might involve isolating your biceps with dumbbell curls. While this can build muscle, it doesn't necessarily translate into practical strength. In contrast, a calisthenics exercise like a pull-up engages not just your biceps but also your shoulders, back, and core, making it a more effective way to build strength that you can use in real-life situations—whether you're lifting a heavy box, climbing a flight of stairs, or playing with your kids.

FLEXIBILITY AND MOBILITY

Another key benefit of calisthenics is that it naturally incorporates flexibility and mobility into your workout routine. Many calisthenics exercises involve a full range of motion, which helps improve joint flexibility and reduce the risk of injury. For instance, deep squats and lunges not only strengthen your legs but also stretch your hip flexors, hamstrings, and calves, promoting better flexibility.

In contrast, traditional gym workouts often focus on lifting heavy weights, sometimes at the expense of flexibility. Over time, this can lead to muscle imbalances and a decrease in range of motion. Calisthenics, on the other hand, promotes balanced muscle development and joint health, making it an excellent choice for long-term fitness.

MENTAL TOUGHNESS AND DISCIPLINE

Calisthenics is as much a mental challenge as it is a physical one. When you're relying solely on your body weight, there's no cheating—no way to lighten the load or take shortcuts. This requires a high level of mental toughness and discipline as you push through the discomfort and keep challenging yourself to reach new levels of strength and endurance.

In the gym, it's easy to get distracted by the environment, the equipment, or even other people. With calisthenics, you learn to focus inward, tuning into your body and your own progress. This mental focus and determination can translate into other areas of your life, helping you develop greater resilience, confidence, and self-control.

WHO IS THIS BOOK FOR?

THIS BOOK IS FOR MEN WHO ARE READY TO TAKE CONTROL OF THEIR FITNESS JOURNEY AND ACHIEVE RESULTS THEY NEVER THOUGHT POSSIBLE. WHETHER YOU'RE A BEGINNER LOOKING TO GET IN SHAPE, AN EXPERIENCED ATHLETE SEEKING A NEW CHALLENGE, OR SOMEONE WHO'S TIRED OF THE TRADITIONAL GYM SCENE, THIS BOOK WILL GUIDE YOU EVERY STEP OF THE WAY.

BEGINNERS LOOKING TO GET IN SHAPE

If you're new to fitness, calisthenics is the perfect starting point. You don't need any prior experience, and you can start with the basics—push-ups, squats, planks, and more. As you progress, you'll build a solid foundation of strength, endurance, and flexibility that will prepare you for more advanced exercises.

This book will walk you through everything you need to know, from proper form and technique to creating a balanced workout routine. You'll learn how to set realistic goals, track your progress, and stay motivated, even when the going gets tough.

EXPERIENCED ATHLETES SEEKING A NEW CHALLENGE

If you're already in good shape but feel like you've hit a plateau with your current workout routine, calisthenics offers a new and exciting challenge. Advanced calisthenics exercises, such as muscle-ups, handstand push-ups, and planches, require a high level of strength, balance, and coordination. Mastering these moves will push your body to its limits and help you achieve new levels of fitness.

This book will provide you with advanced training techniques, tips for breaking through plateaus, and strategies for continuously challenging yourself as you progress. Whether you're training for a specific sport, preparing for a competition, or simply looking to elevate your fitness game, calisthenics will keep you engaged and motivated.

BUSY PROFESSIONALS AND DADS ON THE GO

Life can be hectic, and finding time to work out can be a challenge. If you're a busy professional or a dad with a packed schedule, calisthenics is the perfect solution. You can perform these exercises anywhere, anytime, with minimal equipment and no need to travel to a gym. This book will show you how to fit effective workouts into your busy day, whether you have 10 minutes or an hour to spare.

You'll learn time-efficient routines that target all major muscle groups so you can get a full-body workout in less time. You'll also discover ways to stay active throughout the day, whether you're at home, at work, or on the go. By incorporating calisthenics into your routine, you'll not only stay fit but also have more energy and stamina to tackle whatever life throws at you.

THE BENEFITS OF BODYWEIGHT TRAINING FOR MEN

BODYWEIGHT TRAINING, OR CALISTHENICS, OFFERS A HOST OF BENEFITS SPECIFICALLY TAILORED TO MEN'S FITNESS NEEDS. WHETHER YOUR GOAL IS TO BUILD MUSCLE, IMPROVE ENDURANCE, OR SIMPLY MAINTAIN A HEALTHY LIFESTYLE, CALISTHENICS HAS YOU COVERED.

MUSCLE BUILDING AND STRENGTH GAINS

One of the most common misconceptions about bodyweight training is that it can't build muscle as effectively as weightlifting. This couldn't be further from the truth. When done correctly, calisthenics exercises can lead to significant muscle hypertrophy (growth), especially when you incorporate progressive overload—gradually increasing the difficulty of exercises as you get stronger.

For example, once you've mastered the standard push-up, you can progress to more challenging variations like the archer push-up or the one-arm push-up. These advanced moves place greater demands on your muscles, leading to increased strength and size. Similarly, exercises like pull-ups, dips, and pistol squats target multiple muscle groups at once, promoting balanced muscle development and functional strength.

IMPROVED CARDIOVASCULAR HEALTH

Calisthenics isn't just about building muscle—it's also a great way to improve your cardiovascular health. Many calisthenics exercises are dynamic and involve large muscle groups, which increases your heart rate and burns calories. This makes calisthenics an excellent form of cardio, helping you improve your endurance, burn fat, and keep your heart healthy.

High-intensity calisthenics circuits, where you perform a series of exercises with minimal rest in between, can be particularly effective for cardiovascular conditioning. These workouts not only boost your heart health but also improve your metabolism, making it easier to maintain a lean physique.

ENHANCED FLEXIBILITY AND MOBILITY

As men age, flexibility and mobility often decline, leading to stiffness, reduced range of motion, and an increased risk of injury. Calisthenics addresses this by incorporating movements that promote flexibility and joint health. Exercises like lunges, squats, and hip bridges stretch and strengthen the muscles around your joints, improving your overall flexibility and reducing the risk of injury.

Incorporating regular calisthenics into your routine can help you maintain or even improve your flexibility and mobility, keeping you agile and pain-free as you age. This is especially important for men who want to stay active and enjoy their favorite sports or activities well into their later years.

MENTAL HEALTH AND STRESS RELIEF

Exercise is a powerful tool for managing stress and improving mental health, and calisthenics is no exception. The physical demands of calisthenics require focus, determination, and discipline, which can help clear your mind and reduce stress. The sense of accomplishment that comes from mastering a new exercise or completing a challenging workout can also boost your mood and self-esteem.

Moreover, calisthenics can be a form of meditation in motion. When you're fully engaged in your workout, you're present in the moment, focusing on your breath, your movements, and your body's sensations. This mindfulness can help you disconnect from the stresses of daily life and find a sense of calm and clarity.

LONGEVITY AND QUALITY OF LIFE

Finally, one of the most compelling reasons to choose calisthenics is its impact on longevity and quality of life. Regular calisthenics training can help you maintain a healthy weight, build and preserve muscle mass, improve your cardiovascular health, and reduce the risk of chronic diseases like diabetes and heart disease. By keeping your body strong, flexible, and resilient, you'll be better equipped to enjoy a long, active, and fulfilling life.

MOVING ON

TO SUM IT UP, CALISTHENICS IS MORE THAN JUST A WORKOUT—IT'S A LIFESTYLE THAT CAN TRANSFORM YOUR BODY, MIND, AND SPIRIT. THIS BOOK IS YOUR GUIDE TO MASTERING THE ART OF BODYWEIGHT TRAINING, OFFERING YOU EVERYTHING YOU NEED TO ACHIEVE YOUR FITNESS GOALS AND LIVE A HEALTHIER, MORE VIBRANT LIFE. WHETHER YOU'RE JUST STARTING OUT OR LOOKING TO TAKE YOUR FITNESS TO THE NEXT LEVEL, CALISTHENICS IS THE KEY TO UNLOCKING YOUR FULL POTENTIAL. SO, LET'S GET STARTED ON THIS JOURNEY TOGETHER AND DISCOVER THE INCREDIBLE POWER OF YOUR OWN BODY.

UNDERSTANDING THE FUNDAMENTALS OF CALISTHENICS

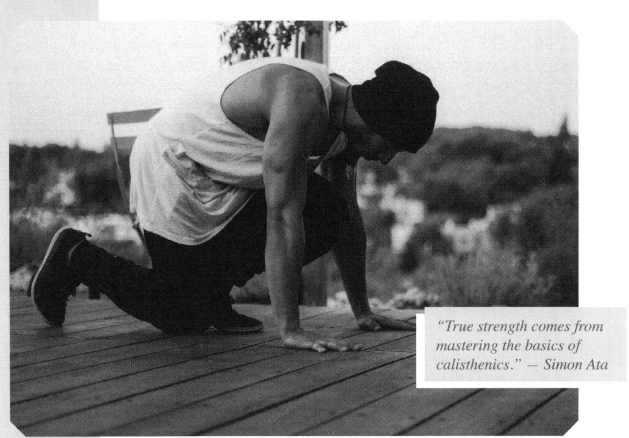

"True strength comes from mastering the basics of calisthenics." — Simon Ata

Imagine waking up every morning with a sense of strength and control over your body that you haven't felt in years. You move through your day with ease, confident in your ability to handle whatever comes your way, whether it's lifting your kids, climbing stairs without a second thought, or simply feeling good in your skin. This is the promise of calisthenics—an age-old practice that reconnects you with the raw, functional strength of your body. Unlike conventional fitness methods that often isolate muscles and focus on aesthetics, calisthenics takes you back to basics, helping you build a body that's not just strong but also capable, flexible, and resilient. But why does this matter to you? Because calisthenics is more than just a workout; it's a journey of mastering your body, gaining control, and enhancing the quality of your everyday life.

In this chapter, we'll explore the philosophy that underpins calisthenics, the science that makes it effective, and the practical benefits it brings to your daily activities. You'll also learn to distinguish between the myths and facts surrounding this form of exercise, arming yourself with the knowledge to make informed decisions about your fitness journey.

THE PHILOSOPHY OF CALISTHENICS: STRENGTH, CONTROL, AND FUNCTIONALITY

AT ITS CORE, CALISTHENICS IS ABOUT MASTERING YOUR OWN BODY. UNLIKE TRADITIONAL WEIGHTLIFTING, WHICH OFTEN FOCUSES ON ISOLATING SPECIFIC MUSCLES TO INCREASE MASS, CALISTHENICS EMPHASIZES THE HARMONIOUS FUNCTIONING OF YOUR ENTIRE BODY. THE PHILOSOPHY BEHIND CALISTHENICS IS ROOTED IN THE IDEA THAT TRUE STRENGTH COMES FROM BEING ABLE TO CONTROL AND MOVE YOUR BODY EFFICIENTLY AND EFFECTIVELY, NO MATTER THE SITUATION.

STRENGTH THROUGH CONTROL

When you think of strength, you might picture someone lifting heavy weights at the gym. While this certainly demonstrates a form of strength, it's not the only kind—or even the most practical. Calisthenics teaches that real strength comes from being able to control your body through a full range of motion. Whether it's performing a perfect pull-up, holding a plank, or executing a deep squat, the focus is on moving with precision and control.

Imagine the strength required to execute a perfect handstand or pull-up. It's not just raw power; it's a blend of balance, coordination, and muscle control. Calisthenics teaches you to engage your entire body as a cohesive unit rather than isolating individual muscles. This holistic approach not only builds physical strength but also enhances your mind-body connection, making you more aware of how your body moves and functions.

This approach to strength is not just about how much you can lift or how big your muscles are. It's about how well you can use your body in real-life situations. For example, being able to lift a heavy box from the ground without injuring yourself, or having the endurance to climb several flights of stairs without getting winded. This is functional strength, and it's the foundation of calisthenics.

FUNCTIONALITY: TRAINING FOR LIFE, NOT JUST THE GYM

One of the core philosophies of calisthenics is functionality. While traditional weightlifting might make you stronger in the gym, calisthenics aims to make you stronger in life. Functional training refers to exercises that mimic real-life movements, improving your ability to perform everyday tasks with ease.

Consider the difference between a bicep curl and a pull-up. While the former isolates the bicep muscle, the latter engages multiple muscle groups, including your back, shoulders, core, and arms. The pull-up is a functional movement because it replicates actions you might perform in daily life, such as pulling yourself up over a ledge or lifting a heavy object off the ground.

This focus on functionality makes calisthenics especially valuable. By training with movements that mirror real-world actions, you're not just building muscle; you're improving your overall ability to move through life efficiently and safely. Whether it's carrying groceries, playing with your kids, or simply maintaining your independence as you age, functional strength is a lifelong asset.

HOW CALISTHENICS WORKS: THE SCIENCE OF BODYWEIGHT RESISTANCE

YOU MIGHT WONDER HOW EXERCISES THAT ONLY USE YOUR BODY WEIGHT CAN BE AS EFFECTIVE AS LIFTING WEIGHTS OR USING MACHINES. THE ANSWER LIES IN THE PRINCIPLES OF BODYWEIGHT RESISTANCE AND THE WAY CALISTHENICS LEVERAGES THESE PRINCIPLES TO BUILD STRENGTH, ENDURANCE, AND FLEXIBILITY.

THE POWER OF BODYWEIGHT EXERCISES

Bodyweight exercises are unique because they require you to move your entire body in space rather than just lifting an external weight. This means that every calisthenic exercise engages multiple muscle groups at once, leading to more efficient workouts and more balanced muscle development.

For instance, a push-up isn't just about your chest and arms; it also engages your core, shoulders, and even your legs to some extent. This integrated approach ensures that no part of your body is left behind, helping you develop a well-rounded physique.

PROGRESSIVE OVERLOAD IN CALISTHENICS

One of the key concepts in strength training is progressive overload, which means gradually increasing the resistance or difficulty of exercises to continue making gains in strength and muscle size. Traditional weightlifting usually involves adding more weight to the bar. However, in calisthenics, progressive overload is achieved by manipulating leverage, increasing the range of motion, or adding explosive movements.

For example, once you've mastered standard push-ups, you can progress to more challenging variations like decline push-ups, archer push-ups, or even one-arm push-ups. Each of these variations increases the difficulty by changing the leverage or requiring greater balance and coordination, thus continuing to challenge your muscles and stimulate growth.

MUSCLE ACTIVATION AND ENDURANCE

In calisthenics, muscle growth occurs primarily through a combination of mechanical tension, metabolic stress, and muscle damage. Mechanical tension is created when you hold or move your body against resistance, such as in a pull-up or plank. Metabolic stress happens when you perform high-repetition exercises that fatigue your muscles, leading to the "pump" feeling that bodybuilders chase. Finally, muscle damage occurs when you push your muscles to their limits, causing microscopic tears that rebuild stronger during recovery.

Studies have shown that bodyweight exercises can activate muscle fibers just as effectively as traditional weight training, especially when performed with proper form and intensity. For instance, a study published in the Journal of Strength and Conditioning Research found that push-ups, when done correctly, can activate the chest muscles to a similar extent as the bench press, a staple weightlifting exercise. This means that you can build significant muscle strength and endurance without needing any equipment at all.

Calisthenics also excels in building muscle endurance, which is the ability of your muscles to sustain repeated contractions over time. This is particularly important for functional fitness, as many everyday activities require sustained effort rather than short bursts of strength. Many exercises, like push-ups or squats, are performed for higher repetitions, challenging your muscles to maintain strength over time. This builds not only muscular endurance but also cardiovascular fitness, making calisthenics a comprehensive workout for both strength and stamina.

FUNCTIONAL MOVEMENTS AND WHY THEY MATTER

FUNCTIONAL MOVEMENTS ARE THE CORNERSTONE OF CALISTHENICS. THESE ARE EXERCISES THAT MIMIC THE NATURAL PATTERNS YOUR BODY GOES THROUGH IN EVERYDAY LIFE, MAKING THEM INCREDIBLY RELEVANT FOR IMPROVING YOUR OVERALL FITNESS AND PREVENTING INJURIES.

THE ROLE OF COMPOUND MOVEMENTS

In calisthenics, most exercises are compound movements, meaning they work multiple muscle groups and joints at the same time. For example, a squat involves your quadriceps, hamstrings, glutes, core, and even your lower back to some extent. This not only makes your workout more efficient but also trains your muscles to work together, as they do in real life.

This contrasts with isolation exercises, like a bicep curl, which only work one muscle at a time. While isolation exercises can be useful for targeting specific muscles, they don't have the same functional benefits as compound movements. By focusing on compound movements, calisthenics helps you build strength in a way that's directly applicable to your daily activities.

THE BENEFITS OF FUNCTIONAL TRAINING

Functional training has several advantages over traditional, muscle-isolating exercises. First, it improves your overall coordination and balance. When you train with functional movements, your muscles learn to work together more effectively, which translates to better performance in real-life activities. This can be particularly beneficial as you age, helping you maintain your independence and reduce the risk of falls or injuries.

Second, functional training enhances your athletic performance. Whether you're a weekend warrior or a professional athlete, training movements that mirror the demands of your sport can improve your agility, speed, and strength. For example, boxers often use push-ups, planks, and pull-ups to develop the upper body strength and core stability needed for powerful punches.

Finally, functional training is time-efficient. Because these exercises engage multiple muscle groups at once, you can get a full-body workout in less time compared to traditional strength training. This makes calisthenics a great option for busy individuals who want to maximize their workout efficiency without sacrificing results.

REAL-LIFE APPLICATIONS OF FUNCTIONAL STRENGTH

The benefits of functional strength extend far beyond the gym. Consider the following scenarios:

*   **Lifting and Carrying:** Whether you're moving boxes, carrying groceries, or lifting your child, functional strength makes these tasks easier and safer. Exercises like squats, deadlifts, and farmer's walks train your body to handle heavy loads with proper form, reducing the risk of injury.

- **Improved Posture:** Many of us spend long hours sitting at a desk, leading to poor posture and back pain. Functional movements like rows, planks, and thoracic rotations can help correct imbalances, strengthen your back muscles, and improve your posture, making those long hours at the computer more comfortable.

- **Everyday Mobility:** Functional training enhances your ability to move through daily life with ease. Whether you're climbing stairs, getting in and out of a car, or simply walking around, functional movements like lunges and step-ups improve your mobility and

flexibility, making these activities feel effortless.

THE IMPORTANCE OF MOBILITY AND FLEXIBILITY

STRENGTH ALONE ISN'T ENOUGH TO ENSURE A HEALTHY, FUNCTIONAL BODY. MOBILITY AND FLEXIBILITY ARE EQUALLY IMPORTANT, AND THEY PLAY A CRUCIAL ROLE IN CALISTHENICS.

DEFINING MOBILITY AND FLEXIBILITY

Mobility refers to the range of motion within a joint, while flexibility refers to the ability of your muscles to stretch. Both are essential for performing calisthenics exercises correctly and safely. Without adequate mobility, you might not be able to achieve the full range of motion in exercises like squats or push-ups, which can limit your progress and increase your risk of injury.

Flexibility, on the other hand, allows your muscles to move freely and without restriction. This is especially important in calisthenics, where many exercises require you to stretch and lengthen your muscles, such as in the case of a deep squat or a back bridge.

THE CONNECTION BETWEEN MOBILITY, FLEXIBILITY, AND STRENGTH

Mobility and flexibility are often overlooked in traditional strength training programs, but in calisthenics, they are given equal importance. This is because, in calisthenics, you need to be able to move your body through a full range of motion to perform exercises correctly. For instance, to do a full push-up, you need good shoulder mobility and chest flexibility. Without these, you might find yourself struggling to complete the exercise, or worse, you could end up injuring yourself.

Moreover, flexibility and mobility contribute to better posture and alignment, which are crucial for preventing injuries and ensuring that your movements are as efficient as possible. By incorporating mobility and flexibility exercises into your calisthenics routine, you're not just building strength—you're also ensuring that your body can move freely and without pain.

PRACTICAL TIPS FOR IMPROVING MOBILITY AND FLEXIBILITY

Improving your mobility and flexibility doesn't have to be complicated. Simple exercises like stretching, yoga, or even dynamic warm-ups before your calisthenics session can make a big difference. For example, hip mobility drills, such as leg swings or deep lunges, can help improve your squat depth, while shoulder dislocations with a resistance band can increase your shoulder mobility, making it easier to perform exercises like push-ups or dips.

Consistency is key when it comes to improving mobility and flexibility. Make these exercises a regular part of your routine, and you'll notice improvements not just in your calisthenics performance, but in how you move and feel every day.

COMMON MYTHS AND MISCONCEPTIONS ABOUT CALISTHENICS

DESPITE ITS MANY BENEFITS, CALISTHENICS IS OFTEN MISUNDERSTOOD OR UNDERESTIMATED. LET'S TAKE A CLOSER LOOK AT SOME OF THE MOST COMMON MYTHS AND MISCONCEPTIONS ABOUT CALISTHENICS AND SET THE RECORD STRAIGHT.

Myth  Calisthenics Can't Build Muscle

One of the most pervasive myths about calisthenics is that it can't build as much muscle as weightlifting. This misconception likely arises from the idea that lifting heavy weights is the only way to achieve hypertrophy (muscle growth). However, calisthenics can be just as effective, if not more so, at building muscle, particularly when combined with progressive overload and proper nutrition.

As mentioned earlier, calisthenics relies on bodyweight resistance, which can be incredibly challenging. Exercises like pull-ups, dips, and push-ups can build significant muscle mass, especially when you progress to more advanced variations. For instance, moving from a regular pull-up to a one-arm pull-up or from a standard push-up to a planche push-up dramatically increases the resistance, stimulating muscle growth.

In fact, many calisthenics athletes boast impressive physiques, proving that you don't need to lift heavy weights to build a muscular body. The key is to continuously challenge your muscles by increasing the difficulty of your exercises, ensuring that you're always working towards new goals.

Myth Calisthenics Is Only for Beginners

Another common misconception is that calisthenics is only for beginners or people who are out of shape. While calisthenics is indeed a great way to get started with fitness, it's also a highly advanced form of training that can challenge even the most experienced athletes.

Advanced calisthenics exercises, like muscle-ups, planches, and handstand push-ups, require immense strength, control, and coordination. These movements take years of dedicated practice to master, making calisthenics a lifelong journey for those who are truly committed.

Myth Calisthenics Is Only for Young, Fit People

Another common misconception is that calisthenics is only suitable for young, fit individuals who are already in good shape. This couldn't be further from the truth. Calisthenics is incredibly versatile and can be adapted to any fitness level, making it accessible to everyone, regardless of age or physical condition.

For beginners or those with limited mobility, calisthenics offers a gentle introduction to exercise, with simple movements like wall push-ups, assisted squats, and plank variations. As you build strength and confidence, you can gradually progress to more challenging exercises, tailoring your workout to your abilities.

For older adults, calisthenics provides a safe and effective way to maintain muscle mass, improve balance, and enhance flexibility—all of which are crucial for healthy aging. By focusing on functional movements and body control, calisthenics helps you stay active and independent as you age, reducing the risk of falls and other injuries.

Myth You Need Equipment to Get a Good Workout

One of the biggest advantages of calisthenics is that you don't need any equipment to get a great workout. All you need is your body and a little bit of space. This makes calisthenics one of the most accessible forms of exercise, as you can do it anywhere, anytime.

That said, you can certainly add equipment like pull-up bars, parallettes, or resistance bands to your calisthenics routine if you want to increase the difficulty or add variety. But even without any equipment, you can still achieve a high level of fitness with calisthenics.

Myth  Calisthenics Is Not as Effective as Weightlifting

Some people believe that calisthenics isn't as effective as weightlifting when it comes to building strength. While it's true that lifting heavy weights can help you build brute strength, calisthenics focuses on a different kind of strength—one that's more functional and transferable to real-life situations.

Calisthenics exercises challenge you to control your body in space, often in ways that weightlifting doesn't. For example, holding a handstand requires immense strength, balance, and coordination—qualities that aren't necessarily developed through traditional weightlifting. Similarly, exercises like muscle-ups, pistol squats, and human flags demand a high level of strength and control that's difficult to achieve with weights alone.

In fact, many elite athletes and military personnel use calisthenics as part of their training because it builds the kind of strength that's practical and applicable to their daily tasks. Whether you're a firefighter, soldier, or simply someone who wants to move better in daily life, calisthenics offers a unique and effective way to build real-world strength.

Myth Calisthenics Is Boring

Finally, some people think that calisthenics is boring or repetitive. This couldn't be further from the truth. The beauty of calisthenics is that it offers endless possibilities for creativity and progression. With so many variations and progressions available for each exercise, you'll never run out of new challenges to keep your workouts fresh and exciting.

Plus, because calisthenics is so versatile, you can tailor your workouts to your personal preferences and goals. Whether you want to focus on strength, endurance, mobility, or flexibility, calisthenics has something to offer.

THE BOTTOM LINE

As you can see, calisthenics is much more than just a workout routine. It's a holistic approach to fitness that emphasizes strength, control, functionality, and mobility. By mastering your own body weight, you're not just building muscle—you're building a body that moves well, feels good, and is capable of handling anything life throws at you.

Whether you're a complete beginner or an experienced athlete, calisthenics has something to offer. It's a journey that will challenge you, inspire you, and ultimately transform your body and your life. So, why not take the first step today? Embrace the philosophy of calisthenics, and discover what your body is truly capable of.

PREPARING
FOR SUCCESS

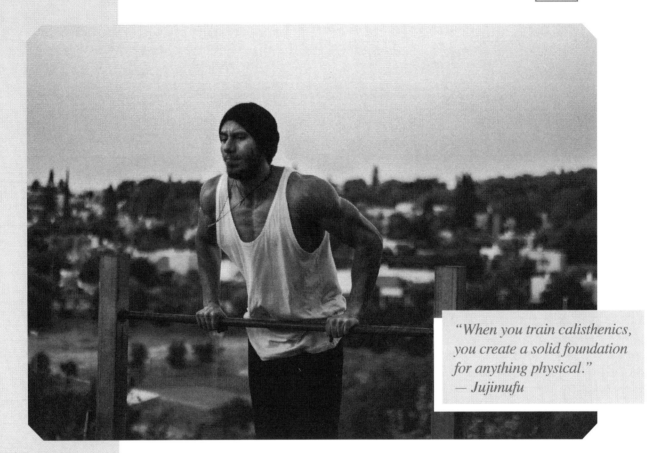

"When you train calisthenics, you create a solid foundation for anything physical."
— *Jujimufu*

Embarking on a fitness journey can feel overwhelming, especially when you're not sure where to start. Whether you're aiming to build muscle, improve endurance, or master advanced calisthenics, the key to success lies in preparation. You wouldn't set off on a road trip without a map or GPS, would you? The same principle applies to your fitness goals. Without a clear plan, it's easy to get lost, lose motivation, or fail to see the progress you desire. This chapter is your guide to preparing for success, helping you set realistic goals, track your progress, and structure your workouts in a way that aligns with your objectives. By the end of this chapter, you'll be equipped with the tools and knowledge needed to start your journey on the right foot, making your goals not just attainable but sustainable.

SETTING REALISTIC GOALS: SHORT-TERM VS. LONG-TERM OBJECTIVES

WHEN IT COMES TO FITNESS, SETTING GOALS IS NOT JUST ABOUT KNOWING WHERE YOU WANT TO GO—IT'S ABOUT CREATING A ROADMAP TO GET THERE. GOALS GIVE YOU DIRECTION, MOTIVATION, AND A WAY TO MEASURE YOUR PROGRESS. HOWEVER, NOT ALL GOALS ARE CREATED EQUAL. TO TRULY SET YOURSELF UP FOR SUCCESS, YOU NEED TO DISTINGUISH BETWEEN SHORT-TERM AND LONG-TERM OBJECTIVES.

- **Short-Term Goals:** These are the stepping stones toward your bigger ambitions. Short-term goals are typically things you can achieve within a few weeks or months. For instance, if your long-term goal is to do ten pull-ups, a short-term goal might be to perform one or two unassisted pull-ups within the next month. These smaller, more immediate targets keep you motivated by providing regular milestones to celebrate.

- **Long-Term Goals:** Long-term goals are your big-picture aspirations. They could be anything from running a marathon to achieving a specific body composition or mastering a complex calisthenics move like the muscle-up. These goals usually take several months to years to achieve and require consistent effort and dedication. While they might seem daunting at first, breaking them down into smaller short-term goals can make them feel more manageable.

Balancing short-term and long-term goals is crucial for maintaining motivation and seeing consistent progress. Short-term goals give you something to celebrate along the way, providing a sense of achievement and encouraging you to keep pushing forward. Long-term goals, meanwhile, keep you focused on the bigger picture, ensuring that all your short-term efforts are leading you toward a meaningful outcome.

SMART GOALS: A FRAMEWORK FOR SUCCESS

To make sure your goals are both realistic and achievable, consider using the SMART criteria. SMART stands for Specific, Measurable, Achievable, Relevant, and Time-bound. This framework helps you clarify your goals, ensuring that they are well-defined and actionable.

- **Specific:** Your goal should be clear and specific. Instead of saying, "I want to get fit," say, "I want to be able to do 20 push-ups in a row."

- **Measurable:** You need to be able to track your progress. Measurable goals allow you to see how far you've come. For example, "I want to reduce my body fat percentage by 5%."

- **Achievable:** While it's great to aim high, your goals should be realistic. If you're new to exercise, aiming to run a marathon in three months might not be feasible. Start with a goal that's challenging but attainable.

- **Relevant:** Your goals should align with your broader objectives. Ask yourself, "Does this goal matter to me?" If you're passionate about strength training, focusing on running might not be the most relevant goal.

- **Time-bound:** Set a deadline for your goal. Having a timeframe creates a sense of urgency and helps you stay focused. For instance, "I want to increase my squat weight by 10 pounds within the next 8 weeks."

One common pitfall in goal setting is being too ambitious. It's great to have big dreams, but if your goals are unrealistic, you might end up feeling discouraged when you don't achieve them as quickly as you'd hoped. Another mistake is not revisiting your goals regularly. As you progress, your goals should evolve to reflect your new fitness level and interests. Make it a habit to review and adjust your goals every few months to ensure they remain challenging yet achievable.

According to James Clear, author of Atomic Habits, "The most effective way to achieve long-term fitness goals is to focus on small, consistent actions that compound over time." This means that instead of trying to make drastic changes overnight, you should focus on making small improvements each day. Over time, these small changes will add up, leading to significant progress.

HOW TO TRACK YOUR PROGRESS: MEASUREMENTS, JOURNALS, AND PHOTOS

TRACKING YOUR PROGRESS IS LIKE KEEPING A JOURNAL OF YOUR JOURNEY. IT NOT ONLY ALLOWS YOU TO SEE HOW FAR YOU'VE COME, BUT IT ALSO HELPS YOU STAY MOTIVATED AND MAKE NECESSARY ADJUSTMENTS TO YOUR PLAN. WITHOUT TRACKING, IT'S EASY TO LOSE SIGHT OF YOUR PROGRESS, WHICH CAN LEAD TO FRUSTRATION AND A SENSE OF STAGNATION. WHEN YOU TRACK YOUR PROGRESS, YOU CAN IDENTIFY WHAT'S WORKING AND WHAT'S NOT AND MAKE INFORMED DECISIONS MOVING FORWARD.

DIFFERENT METHODS OF TRACKING PROGRESS

There are several effective ways to track your progress, each offering unique insights into your journey. You might choose to use one method or combine several, depending on your goals and preferences.

- **Measurements:** Tracking measurements is particularly useful if your goals are related to body composition changes. Key measurements to track include your waist, hips, chest, arms, and thighs. Measuring yourself regularly—every two weeks, for example—can provide a more accurate picture of your progress than simply relying on the scale. Remember, muscle weighs more than fat, so even if the scale doesn't budge, you might still be losing inches.

- **Journals:** A fitness journal is a powerful tool for tracking not just your physical progress but also your thoughts, feelings, and experiences along the way. In your journal, you can record your workouts, noting the exercises you performed, the number of sets and reps, and how you felt during and after the session. You can also use your journal to document your nutrition, sleep patterns, and any challenges or successes you encounter. Over time, your journal becomes a valuable resource that helps you understand what works best for you.

- **Photos:** Progress photos offer a visual representation of your transformation. While it can be difficult to notice changes in the mirror day-to-day, comparing photos taken weeks or months apart can highlight significant progress. To get the most accurate comparison, take your photos in the same lighting, at the same time of day, and in similar clothing. You might feel self-conscious at first, but these photos can be incredibly motivating as you start to see the changes in your body.

While each of these methods can be effective on its own, combining them gives you a more comprehensive view of your progress. For example, you might notice that your weight hasn't changed much, but your measurements show a decrease in body fat, and your progress photos reveal more muscle definition. Together, these indicators provide a fuller picture of your progress and help you stay motivated.

Tracking your progress can sometimes feel tedious, especially if you're not seeing immediate results. However, it's important to remember that progress in fitness is often slow and incremental. Even small improvements should be celebrated, as they indicate that you're moving in the right direction.

ASSESSING YOUR CURRENT FITNESS LEVEL

BEFORE YOU CAN CREATE AN EFFECTIVE WORKOUT PLAN, YOU NEED TO KNOW WHERE YOU'RE STARTING FROM. ASSESSING YOUR CURRENT FITNESS LEVEL GIVES YOU A BASELINE TO WORK FROM AND HELPS YOU SET REALISTIC GOALS. IT ALSO ALLOWS YOU TO TAILOR YOUR WORKOUTS TO YOUR SPECIFIC NEEDS, ENSURING THAT YOU'RE NOT OVEREXERTING YOURSELF OR, CONVERSELY, NOT CHALLENGING YOURSELF ENOUGH.

HOW TO PERFORM A BASIC FITNESS ASSESSMENT

A comprehensive fitness assessment should evaluate several key areas: cardiovascular endurance, muscular strength, muscular endurance, flexibility, and body composition. Here's how you can assess each area:

- **Cardiovascular Endurance:** To assess your cardiovascular endurance, perform a simple test like the 1-mile walk or run. Time yourself and note how long it takes to complete the distance. If you're walking, note your heart rate immediately after finishing. As you progress, aim to reduce your time or lower your heart rate after the same effort.

- **Muscular Strength:** You can assess your muscular strength with exercises like push-ups, squats, or planks. For push-ups, see how many you can perform with good form before reaching fatigue. The same goes for squats. For planks, time how long you can hold the position without your form breaking down.

- **Flexibility:** Flexibility is often overlooked, but it's crucial for overall fitness and injury prevention. A simple way to assess your flexibility is the sit-and-reach test. Sit on the floor with your legs straight out in front of you. Reach forward as far as you can, keeping your legs straight. Measure the distance between your fingertips and your toes.

- **Body Composition:** While body composition is more challenging to measure at home, you can estimate it with tools like a tape measure or a simple body fat caliper. For a more accurate assessment, you might consider visiting a fitness professional who can use more advanced tools like bioelectrical impedance analysis (BIA) or dual-energy X-ray absorptiometry (DEXA).

INTERPRETING YOUR RESULTS

Once you've completed your assessment, it's time to interpret your results. Compare your performance to standard benchmarks for your age and gender, which you can find online or in fitness resources. If you fall below average in a particular area, that's a sign that it might need more attention in your training plan. Conversely, if you excel in another area, you might choose to set more challenging goals for yourself in that domain.

You can also interpret the results in the context of your goals. For example, if your goal is to build muscle, your focus should be on improving your muscular strength and endurance. If your goal is to improve cardiovascular health, you'll want to focus on improving your run or walk time. Use your assessment results to guide your workout plan and set specific goals for improvement.

HOW TO STRUCTURE YOUR WORKOUTS BASED ON YOUR GOALS

NOT ALL WORKOUTS ARE CREATED EQUAL, AND WHAT WORKS FOR ONE PERSON MIGHT NOT WORK FOR ANOTHER. THE KEY TO SUCCESS IS STRUCTURING YOUR WORKOUTS TO ALIGN WITH YOUR SPECIFIC GOALS. WHETHER YOU WANT TO BUILD MUSCLE, IMPROVE ENDURANCE, OR MASTER CALISTHENICS SKILLS, YOUR WORKOUT PLAN SHOULD BE TAILORED TO HELP YOU ACHIEVE THOSE OBJECTIVES.

BUILDING MUSCLE

If your primary goal is to build muscle, your workout plan should focus on resistance training. This involves lifting weights, using resistance bands, or performing bodyweight exercises that challenge your muscles. Aim for compound movements like squats, deadlifts, and bench presses, which work multiple muscle groups simultaneously and promote overall strength and muscle growth.

- **Reps and Sets:** For muscle growth, focus on lifting heavier weights with fewer repetitions. A typical hypertrophy workout might involve 3-4 sets of 8-12 reps for each exercise. It's important to challenge yourself, but always maintain good form to avoid injury.

- **Rest Periods:** Between sets, take a short rest period—typically 60-90 seconds. This allows your muscles to recover just enough to perform the next set with good form while still maintaining the intensity needed for muscle growth.

- **Progressive Overload:** To continue building muscle, you need to progressively increase the weight you're lifting or the difficulty of the exercises you're performing. This concept, known as progressive overload, ensures that your muscles are continually challenged and continue to grow over time.

IMPROVING ENDURANCE

If your goal is to improve endurance, your workout plan should focus on activities that increase your cardiovascular fitness. This might include running, cycling, swimming, or high-intensity interval training (HIIT).

- **Cardio Workouts:** For endurance, aim for longer, steady-state cardio sessions. For example, you might start with a 30-minute run at a moderate pace and gradually increase the duration as your endurance improves. If you prefer variety, cycling or swimming can provide a similar cardiovascular challenge.

- HIIT: High-Intensity Interval Training (HIIT) is another effective way to build endurance. HIIT involves short bursts of intense exercise followed by periods of rest or lower-intensity exercise. For example, you might sprint for 30 seconds, then walk or jog for 1-2 minutes, and repeat for a total of 20-30 minutes. HIIT is particularly effective because it not only improves endurance but also burns a significant number of calories in a short amount of time.

- Strength Training for Endurance: While cardio is crucial for endurance, don't neglect strength training. Incorporating lighter weights and higher repetitions into your strength routine can enhance muscular endurance, making it easier to maintain good form and power through longer workouts.

MASTERING CALISTHENICS SKILLS

For those interested in mastering advanced calisthenics skills like the muscle-up, handstand, or human flag, your workout plan needs to be focused on building the specific strength and technique required for these movements.

- Skill-Specific Training: Start by breaking down each skill into its component parts. For example, to master the muscle-up, you'll need to develop strength in both the pull-up and the dip. Practice these movements separately before attempting the full skill. Use resistance bands to assist with difficult portions of the movement as you build strength.

- Progressions: Progressions are key to mastering calisthenics skills. This means starting with easier variations of a movement and gradually increasing the difficulty as your strength and technique improve. For example, if you're working on handstands, start with wall-assisted handstands before moving on to freestanding handstands.

- Consistency: Consistency is crucial when working on skill-based movements. Practice the specific skills you want to master multiple times per week. Even 10-15 minutes of focused practice can make a big difference over time.

No matter what your goals are, it's important to balance the intensity of your workouts with adequate recovery. Overtraining can lead to burnout, injury, and decreased performance, so make sure to include rest days in your plan. Active recovery, such as light cardio or stretching, can help promote blood flow and aid in muscle recovery without putting too much strain on your body.

ESSENTIAL GEAR: MINIMAL EQUIPMENT FOR MAXIMUM RESULTS

ONE OF THE GREAT THINGS ABOUT CALISTHENICS IS THAT YOU DON'T NEED A GYM FULL OF EQUIPMENT TO GET IN SHAPE. IN FACT, YOU CAN ACHIEVE INCREDIBLE RESULTS WITH MINIMAL GEAR, MAKING IT A COST-EFFECTIVE AND CONVENIENT OPTION FOR ANYONE LOOKING TO IMPROVE THEIR FITNESS. HOWEVER, INVESTING IN A FEW KEY PIECES OF EQUIPMENT CAN ENHANCE YOUR WORKOUTS AND HELP YOU ACHIEVE YOUR GOALS MORE EFFICIENTLY.

PULL-UP BARS

A pull-up bar is one of the most versatile pieces of equipment you can own. It allows you to perform a wide range of exercises, from standard pull-ups to more advanced moves like muscle-ups or hanging leg raises. Pull-up bars come in various forms, from door-mounted options to freestanding units that can be placed anywhere in your home.

- **Benefits of Pull-Up Bars:** Pull-up bars target your back, shoulders, arms, and core, making them essential for building upper body strength. They're particularly effective for those focusing on calisthenics, as many advanced movements, such as the muscle-up or front lever, require a strong pull-up foundation.

- **Types of Pull-Up Bars:** If space is an issue, a door-mounted pull-up bar is a great option. These are easy to install and remove, making them ideal for home use. For more versatility, consider a freestanding pull-up bar, which offers additional stability and the ability to perform a wider range of exercises.

RESISTANCE BANDS

Resistance bands are another excellent addition to your home gym. They're lightweight, portable, and incredibly versatile, allowing you to perform a wide variety of exercises that target different muscle groups.

- **Benefits of Resistance Bands:** Resistance bands are ideal for both strength training and stretching. They provide variable resistance, which means the resistance increases as the band stretches, offering a unique challenge compared to free weights. This makes them perfect for working on progressive overload and building strength.

- **Using Resistance Bands:** Resistance bands can be used to modify traditional exercises or create entirely new ones. For example, you can use a resistance band to assist with pull-ups if you're not yet able to perform them unassisted. They're also great for adding resistance to bodyweight exercises like squats or push-ups, making them more challenging and effective.

OTHER ESSENTIAL GEAR

While pull-up bars and resistance bands are often the most recommended, there are a few other pieces of equipment that can enhance your calisthenics workouts.

- **Gymnastic Rings:** Gymnastic rings offer a new level of challenge and versatility. They're great for building upper body and core strength and can be used for a wide range of exercises, from ring rows to ring dips and even muscle-ups.

- **Parallettes:** Parallettes are small, portable bars that allow you to perform exercises like push-ups, L-sits, and planche progressions with greater ease and range of motion. They're particularly useful for those working on advanced calisthenics skills.

- **Jump Rope:** A jump rope is a simple but highly effective tool for improving cardiovascular fitness and coordination. It's also a great way to warm up before your workout or add some high-intensity interval training to your routine.

Even with minimal equipment, you can create a highly effective workout routine that targets all areas of fitness. For example, a simple pull-up bar can be used for a full upper body workout, while resistance bands can be used to add variety and challenge to your leg and core exercises. By incorporating these tools into your routine, you can enhance the effectiveness of your workouts without needing to invest in a lot of expensive equipment.

BRINGING IT ALL TOGETHER: CREATING YOUR PERSONALIZED FITNESS PLAN

NOW THAT YOU UNDERSTAND THE IMPORTANCE OF GOAL SETTING, TRACKING YOUR PROGRESS, ASSESSING YOUR FITNESS LEVEL, STRUCTURING YOUR WORKOUTS, AND USING ESSENTIAL GEAR, IT'S TIME TO BRING IT ALL TOGETHER INTO A PERSONALIZED FITNESS PLAN. YOUR PLAN SHOULD BE TAILORED TO YOUR SPECIFIC GOALS, FITNESS LEVEL, AND LIFESTYLE, ENSURING THAT IT'S BOTH EFFECTIVE AND SUSTAINABLE.

STEP 1 SET YOUR GOALS

Start by setting clear, realistic goals for what you want to achieve. Write down both your short-term and long-term goals, and make sure they're SMART—Specific, Measurable, Achievable, Relevant, and Time-bound.

STEP 2 ASSESS YOUR FITNESS LEVEL

Perform a comprehensive fitness assessment to determine your starting point. Use the results to guide your workout plan, ensuring that you're challenging yourself without overexerting.

STEP 3 STRUCTURE YOUR WORKOUTS

Based on your goals and fitness level, create a workout plan that includes a balance of resistance training, cardiovascular exercise, and flexibility work. Make sure to include rest days and adjust the intensity of your workouts as needed.

STEP 4 TRACK YOUR PROGRESS

Choose the method(s) that work best for you—whether it's taking measurements, keeping a fitness journal, or taking progress photos—and commit to tracking your progress regularly. Use this information to make adjustments to your plan as needed.

STEP 5 USE THE RIGHT EQUIPMENT

Invest in the essential gear that will enhance your workouts, such as a pull-up bar, resistance bands, or gymnastic rings. Use this equipment to add variety and challenge to your routine.

STEP 6 STAY CONSISTENT AND ADJUST AS NEEDED

Consistency is key to success in fitness. Stick to your plan, but also be flexible and willing to make adjustments as you progress. If you're not seeing the results you want, don't be afraid to tweak your plan or try new exercises.

THE BOTTOM LINE

As you prepare to embark on your fitness journey, remember that success is not about perfection; it's about consistency and progress. By setting realistic goals, tracking your progress, assessing your current fitness level, and structuring your workouts effectively, you're laying a strong foundation for long-term success. With minimal equipment and a personalized plan that aligns with your goals, you're well on your way to achieving the results you desire.

Your journey will have its ups and downs, but with the right preparation, you can navigate the challenges and celebrate the victories. Keep your eyes on your goals, stay committed to your plan, and don't be afraid to adjust as needed. The most important thing is that you keep moving forward, one step, one rep, one day at a time.

Now that you've prepared for success, it's time to dive into the next chapter, where we'll explore the fundamentals of nutrition and how to fuel your body for optimal performance. With the right mindset and the tools you've gained in this chapter, you're ready to take the next step in your fitness journey.

THE ROLE OF NUTRITION IN CALISTHENICS

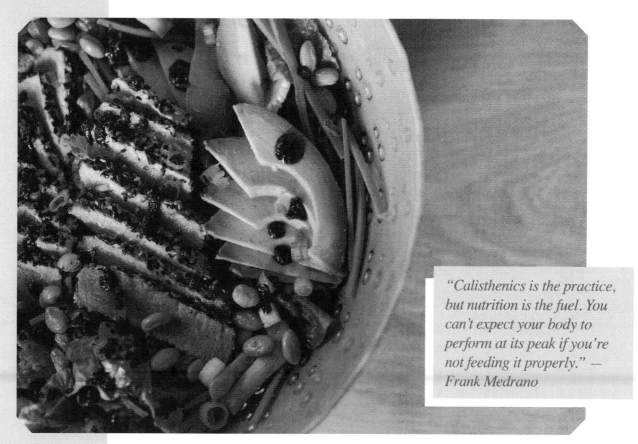

> *"Calisthenics is the practice, but nutrition is the fuel. You can't expect your body to perform at its peak if you're not feeding it properly." — Frank Medrano*

Imagine this: you've just finished an intense calisthenics workout. Your muscles are burning, your heart is racing, and you're drenched in sweat. You've pushed your body to its limits, mastering pull-ups, push-ups, and muscle-ups. But what happens next?

How do you ensure that all your hard work translates into real results? This is where nutrition steps in. No matter how hard you train, your progress will be limited without the right fuel. Proper nutrition isn't just about eating to stay full; it's about giving your body what it needs to recover, build muscle, and stay energized.

Understanding how to fuel your body properly can make all the difference in your calisthenics journey. In this chapter, we'll explore the critical role that nutrition plays in enhancing your performance, speeding up recovery, and helping you achieve your fitness goals.

CALISTHENICS AND THE IMPORTANCE OF DIET

WHEN YOU EMBARK ON YOUR CALISTHENICS JOURNEY, IT'S EASY TO FOCUS SOLELY ON MASTERING THE PERFECT PUSH-UP, PULL-UP, OR HANDSTAND. BUT THERE'S ANOTHER CRITICAL FACTOR THAT CAN MAKE OR BREAK YOUR PROGRESS: YOUR DIET. THINK OF NUTRITION AS THE FOUNDATION UPON WHICH YOUR TRAINING IS BUILT. WITHOUT A STRONG FOUNDATION, EVEN THE MOST WELL-PLANNED WORKOUTS WILL YIELD LIMITED RESULTS.

You might be wondering why diet is so crucial for calisthenics. The answer lies in the unique demands this form of exercise places on your body. Calisthenics, which relies on bodyweight exercises, requires not only strength and endurance but also agility and balance. The right diet fuels your body, allowing you to perform at your best while also aiding in recovery and preventing injury. Whether your goal is to build muscle, lose fat, or simply maintain your current physique, what you eat plays a pivotal role in your success.

Let's dive deeper into how nutrition and calisthenics are interconnected and why what you put on your plate matters just as much as the time you spend training.

UNDERSTANDING MACRONUTRIENTS: PROTEIN, CARBS, AND FATS

WHEN IT COMES TO NUTRITION, MACRONUTRIENTS ARE THE HEAVY HITTERS. TO TRULY OPTIMIZE YOUR DIET FOR CALISTHENICS, YOU MUST UNDERSTAND THE THREE MACRONUTRIENTS: PROTEIN, CARBOHYDRATES, AND FATS. EACH PLAYS A DISTINCT ROLE IN YOUR BODY, AND CORRECTLY BALANCING THEM CAN SIGNIFICANTLY IMPACT YOUR TRAINING OUTCOMES.

PROTEIN: THE MUSCLE REPAIR MECHANIC

Protein is often hailed as the king of macronutrients for anyone serious about fitness, and for good reason. When you perform calisthenics exercises like push-ups, dips, or planks, your muscles undergo stress, causing tiny tears in the muscle fibers. Protein plays a crucial role in repairing these fibers, leading to muscle growth and increased strength over time.

But how much protein do you actually need? The general guideline is to consume around 1.6 to 2.2 grams of protein per kilogram of body weight per day if you're actively training. For someone weighing 70 kilograms (about 154 pounds), this equates to 112 to 154 grams of protein daily. This might seem like a lot, but it's necessary to support muscle repair and growth, especially if you're pushing your body to its limits with calisthenics. Also, according to the American College of Sports Medicine, consuming 20 to 30 grams of protein within 30 minutes after your workout can maximize muscle repair and growth.

Incorporating a variety of protein sources—such as lean meats, fish, eggs, dairy, legumes, and plant-based options like tofu and tempeh—ensures you're getting all the essential amino acids your body needs. Expert nutritionist Dr. John Berardi explains, "Protein intake is fundamental in muscle recovery. Without adequate protein, your body won't be able to repair and rebuild muscle tissue effectively, hindering your progress in any physical training regimen."

CARBOHYDRATES: THE ENERGY POWERHOUSE

Carbohydrates often get a bad rap, especially in the context of weight loss. However, when it comes to calisthenics, carbs are your body's primary energy source, powering you through those intense training sessions.

Carbs are broken down into glucose, which your muscles use as fuel during exercise. If you're doing high-intensity calisthenics workouts, like circuit training or explosive movements, your body needs a steady supply of glucose to maintain performance. Without enough carbs, you might find yourself feeling sluggish, unable to push through those last few reps.

The amount of carbohydrates you need can vary depending on your training intensity and overall goals. For those focusing on muscle gain, consuming around 3 to 6 grams of carbohydrates per kilogram of body weight is recommended. For fat loss, you might reduce this slightly, but it's crucial not to cut carbs too drastically, as they are still vital for maintaining energy levels during your workouts. The International Society of Sports Nutrition recommends that athletes consume 3 to 5 grams of carbohydrates per kilogram of body weight per day to maintain optimal energy levels. Opt for complex carbohydrates like whole grains, sweet potatoes, fruits, and vegetables. These not only provide sustained energy but also come packed with fiber, vitamins, and minerals that support overall health.

FATS: THE UNSUNG HERO

Fats often take a backseat to protein and carbs in fitness discussions, but they play a vital role in maintaining overall health and supporting your calisthenics training. Healthy fats are essential for hormone production, including testosterone, which is crucial for muscle growth and recovery.

Fats also help your body absorb fat-soluble vitamins like A, D, E, and K, which are important for various bodily functions, including immune support and bone health. Additionally, fats provide a concentrated source of energy. While carbohydrates are your body's preferred energy source during high-intensity workouts, fats become more important during longer, lower-intensity activities.

Aim to include healthy fats from sources like avocados, nuts, seeds, olive oil, and fatty fish like salmon in your diet. These foods not only support your training but also contribute to heart health and overall well-being.

In summary, a balanced intake of protein, carbohydrates, and fats is essential for fueling your calisthenics workouts and supporting recovery and growth. As Dr. Berardi emphasizes, "Each macronutrient plays a unique role in your body, and neglecting any one of them can lead to suboptimal performance and recovery."

MICRONUTRIENTS FOR OPTIMAL PERFORMANCE AND RECOVERY

WHILE MACRONUTRIENTS GET MOST OF THE ATTENTION, MICRONUTRIENTS—VITAMINS AND MINERALS—ARE JUST AS IMPORTANT FOR OPTIMAL PERFORMANCE AND RECOVERY IN CALISTHENICS. THESE NUTRIENTS MAY BE REQUIRED IN SMALLER AMOUNTS, BUT THEIR IMPACT ON YOUR BODY'S FUNCTIONING IS SIGNIFICANT.

THE ROLE OF VITAMINS IN CALISTHENICS

Vitamins play a crucial role in energy production, immune function, and muscle recovery. For instance, B vitamins, including B6, B12, and folate, are essential for converting the food you eat into usable energy. They also help in the production of red blood cells, which transport oxygen to your muscles during exercise.

Vitamin D is another critical nutrient, particularly for those engaging in calisthenics. It helps in calcium absorption, which is vital for bone health. Strong bones are essential when you're performing weight-bearing exercises like squats and lunges. Moreover, vitamin D has been linked to improved muscle strength and recovery. However, many people are deficient in this vitamin, especially those living in regions with limited sunlight. Consider getting your vitamin D levels checked and supplementing if necessary.

Antioxidant vitamins, such as vitamins C and E, help protect your body from the oxidative stress that can result from intense exercise. Oxidative stress can lead to muscle damage and delayed recovery, so ensuring adequate intake of these vitamins can help you recover faster and get back to training sooner.

ESSENTIAL MINERALS FOR CALISTHENICS

Minerals are equally important in supporting your calisthenics performance. Calcium, magnesium, and potassium are particularly crucial.

- **Calcium:** Calcium is well-known for its role in bone health, but it's also important for muscle function. It aids in muscle contraction, which is essential when you're performing exercises like push-ups or pull-ups.

- **Magnesium:** Magnesium plays a role in over 300 enzymatic reactions in the body, including those involved in energy production and muscle contraction. It also helps regulate nerve function, which is vital for maintaining the mind-muscle connection during your workouts.

- **Potassium:** Potassium is crucial for maintaining proper fluid balance, nerve signals, and muscle contractions. A deficiency in potassium can lead to muscle cramps and fatigue, hindering your performance.

- **Iron:** Iron is another critical mineral, especially for those engaging in endurance-focused calisthenics routines. Iron is a key component of hemoglobin, the molecule in red blood cells that transports oxygen to your muscles. Without enough iron, your muscles won't get the oxygen they need, leading to fatigue and decreased performance.

- **Zinc:** Zinc is vital for immune function and plays a role in muscle repair and recovery. Intense training can suppress the immune system, making you more susceptible to illness. Ensuring adequate zinc intake can help support your immune system and keep you healthy and training consistently. You can find zinc in foods like meat, shellfish, dairy products, and legumes. If you're not getting enough from your diet, consider a zinc supplement, especially during periods of intense training.

Incorporating a variety of nutrient-dense foods in your diet ensures you get a wide range of micronutrients that support your training, recovery, and overall health. As nutrition expert Dr. Rhonda Patrick notes, "Micronutrients are the foundation of health. Without them, the body cannot function optimally, and this becomes even more apparent when you're pushing your body with intense physical activity."

BUILDING A DIET FOR MUSCLE GROWTH AND FAT LOSS

WHETHER YOU'RE LOOKING TO BUILD MUSCLE, LOSE FAT, OR SIMPLY MAINTAIN YOUR CURRENT PHY-SIQUE, YOUR DIET IS THE KEY TO ACHIEVING THESE GOALS. WHILE THE PRINCIPLES OF HEALTHY EATING REMAIN CONSISTENT, THE WAY YOU ADJUST YOUR MACRONUTRIENT RATIOS AND CALORIC INTAKE WILL VARY DEPENDING ON YOUR OBJECTIVES.

MUSCLE GROWTH: THE CALORIC SURPLUS

To build muscle, you need to be in a caloric surplus, meaning you're consuming more calories than your body burns in a day. This surplus provides the energy your body needs to repair and grow muscle tissue after your calisthenics workouts.

However, this doesn't mean you should start eating anything and everything. The quality of your calories matters just as much as the quantity. Focus on consuming nutrient-dense foods that provide the necessary protein, carbohydrates, and fats, along with a variety of vitamins and minerals.

A good starting point is to increase your daily caloric intake by 250 to 500 calories. This range is typically sufficient to promote muscle growth without excessive fat gain. Adjust your intake based on your progress, increasing or decreasing as needed.

PROTEIN: THE CORNERSTONE OF MUSCLE GROWTH

As mentioned earlier, protein is essential for muscle repair and growth. Aim for a higher protein intake when focusing on muscle building—around 2.2 grams of protein per kilogram of body weight. This increased intake ensures your muscles have the necessary building blocks to recover and grow after each workout.

CARBOHYDRATES: FUELING INTENSE WORKOUTS

Carbohydrates are particularly important when you're in a muscle-building phase. They provide the energy needed for intense calisthenics workouts and help replenish glycogen stores in your muscles. A good rule of thumb is to consume around 4 to 7 grams of carbohydrates per kilogram of body weight, depending on your activity level.

FATS: SUPPORTING HORMONE PRODUCTION

Healthy fats are crucial for hormone production, including testosterone, which plays a significant role in muscle growth. Aim to get around 20-30% of your daily caloric intake from fats, focusing on sources like avocados, nuts, seeds, and olive oil.

FAT LOSS: THE CALORIC DEFICIT

If your goal is to lose fat, you need to create a caloric deficit, meaning you consume fewer calories than your body burns. This deficit forces your body to use stored fat as energy, leading to fat loss over time.

However, it's important not to cut calories too drastically, as this can lead to muscle loss and a decrease in metabolism. A moderate deficit of 500 calories per day is typically sufficient to lose about 0.5 to 1 kilogram (1-2 pounds) of fat per week.

MAINTENANCE: THE CALORIC BALANCE

If your goal is to maintain your current physique, your diet should focus on achieving caloric balance, where your caloric intake matches your caloric expenditure. This allows you to maintain your weight and muscle mass while continuing to improve your calisthenics performance.

Focus on a balanced intake of protein, carbohydrates, and fats, and adjust your portions as needed based on your training intensity and overall activity level.

HYDRATION AND ITS IMPACT ON PERFORMANCE

HYDRATION IS OFTEN OVERLOOKED, BUT IT'S ONE OF THE MOST CRITICAL FACTORS INFLUENCING YOUR CALISTHENICS PERFORMANCE. WATER PLAYS A CRUCIAL ROLE IN NEARLY EVERY BODILY FUNCTION, FROM REGULATING BODY TEMPERATURE TO TRANSPORTING NUTRIENTS AND OXYGEN TO YOUR MUSCLES.

WHEN YOU'RE DEHYDRATED, EVEN SLIGHTLY, YOUR PERFORMANCE CAN SUFFER. YOU MIGHT EXPERIENCE FATIGUE, REDUCED ENDURANCE, AND IMPAIRED COORDINATION—NONE OF WHICH ARE CONDUCIVE TO MASTERING THE DEMANDING MOVEMENTS OF CALISTHENICS.

HOW MUCH WATER DO YOU NEED?

The amount of water you need depends on various factors, including your body weight, climate, and the intensity of your workouts. A general guideline is to aim for 2 to 3 liters (about 8-12 cups) of water per day. However, if you're engaging in intense calisthenics workouts, especially in a hot environment, you may need more.

An easy way to monitor your hydration is by checking the color of your urine. Pale yellow indicates proper hydration, while darker urine suggests you need to drink more water.

ELECTROLYTES: MORE THAN JUST WATER

When you sweat during your workouts, you lose not only water but also electrolytes, which are minerals like sodium, potassium, and magnesium. These electrolytes are vital for muscle function, nerve signaling, and maintaining fluid balance.

Replenishing electrolytes is important, especially after intense training sessions. You can do this by consuming electrolyte-rich foods, such as bananas, nuts, and leafy greens, or by drinking an electrolyte solution if needed.

TIMING YOUR HYDRATION

It's not just about how much you drink but also when you drink. Aim to hydrate consistently throughout the day rather than trying to chug a large amount of water all at once. Drinking water before, during, and after your workouts ensures you stay hydrated and perform at your best.

SAMPLE MEAL PLANS FOR DIFFERENT GOALS

NOW THAT YOU UNDERSTAND THE ROLE OF MACRONUTRIENTS, MICRONUTRIENTS, AND HYDRATION IN SUPPORTING YOUR CALISTHENICS TRAINING, LET'S PUT IT ALL TOGETHER WITH SOME SAMPLE MEAL PLANS TAILORED TO DIFFERENT GOALS. THESE MEAL PLANS ARE DESIGNED TO PROVIDE THE RIGHT BALANCE OF NUTRIENTS TO SUPPORT MUSCLE GAIN, FAT LOSS, OR MAINTENANCE WHILE KEEPING YOUR ENERGY LEVELS HIGH AND YOUR RECOVERY ON TRACK.

SAMPLE MEAL PLAN FOR MUSCLE GAIN

BREAKFAST:
- Oatmeal with a scoop of protein powder, topped with mixed berries and a handful of nuts.
- A glass of milk or a protein shake.

MID-MORNING SNACK:
- Greek yogurt with honey and a banana.
- A handful of almonds.

LUNCH:
- Grilled chicken breast with quinoa and roasted vegetables (broccoli, carrots, bell peppers).
- A side salad with olive oil and balsamic vinegar dressing.

AFTERNOON SNACK:
- A protein bar or a peanut butter sandwich on whole-grain bread.
- An apple.

DINNER:
- Baked salmon with sweet potato and steamed asparagus.
- A mixed green salad with avocado and sunflower seeds.

EVENING SNACK:
- Cottage cheese with a drizzle of honey and a few slices of pineapple.

SAMPLE MEAL PLAN FOR FAT LOSS

BREAKFAST:
- Scrambled eggs with spinach and tomatoes.
- A slice of whole-grain toast.

MID-MORNING SNACK:
- A small handful of mixed nuts.
- An orange or a pear.

LUNCH:
- Grilled turkey breast with a large mixed salad (lettuce, cucumber, cherry tomatoes, bell peppers) topped with olive oil and lemon juice.
- A small serving of brown rice.

AFTERNOON SNACK:
•Carrot and celery sticks with hummus.

DINNER:
•Grilled shrimp with cauliflower rice and sautéed zucchini.
•A side of steamed broccoli.

EVENING SNACK:
•A small bowl of Greek yogurt with a sprinkle of flaxseeds.

SAMPLE MEAL PLAN FOR MAINTENANCE

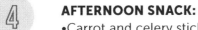

BREAKFAST:
•Smoothie with spinach, banana, almond butter, and a scoop of protein powder.
•A slice of whole-grain toast with avocado.

MID-MORNING SNACK:
•A hard-boiled egg and a handful of cherry tomatoes.

LUNCH:
•Grilled chicken wrap with whole-grain tortilla, lettuce, tomatoes, and avocado.
•A side of fruit, like an apple or a pear.

AFTERNOON SNACK:
•A handful of mixed nuts and dried fruit.

DINNER:
•Grilled beef steak with quinoa and roasted vegetables (carrots, bell peppers, Brussels sprouts).
•A mixed green salad with olive oil and vinegar.

EVENING SNACK:
• A small bowl of cottage cheese with sliced peaches.

These meal plans provide a framework to help you achieve your specific goals. Remember, the key to success is consistency, both in your workouts and your diet. Listen to your body, adjust as needed, and stay committed to your nutrition plan.

THE BOTTOM LINE

In the world of calisthenics, your diet is just as important as your training. Proper nutrition fuels your body, supports recovery, and helps you achieve your fitness goals, whether you're aiming to build muscle, lose fat, or maintain your current physique. By understanding the roles of macronutrients and micronutrients, staying hydrated, and tailoring your diet to your specific needs, you can maximize your performance and get the most out of your calisthenics journey.

Remember, there's no one-size-fits-all approach to nutrition. It's about finding what works best for you, making adjustments along the way, and staying consistent. With the right diet in place, you'll not only see better results in your calisthenics training but also feel stronger, healthier, and more energized every day.

BEGINNER CALISTHENICS EXERCISES

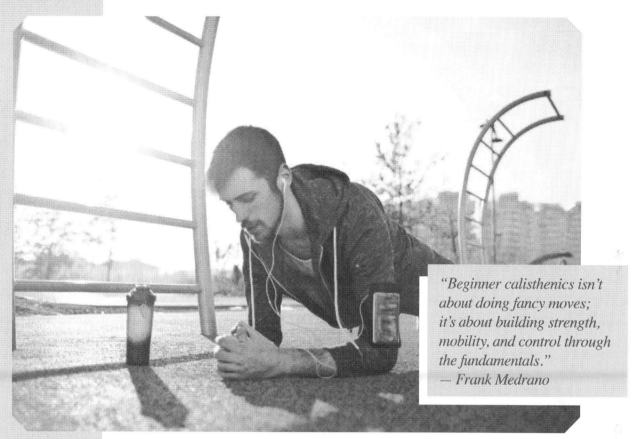

"Beginner calisthenics isn't about doing fancy moves; it's about building strength, mobility, and control through the fundamentals."
— *Frank Medrano*

Starting your fitness journey can feel overwhelming, but calisthenics is an excellent place to begin. Unlike weightlifting or high-intensity workouts, calisthenics uses your body as the primary tool.

This means you can work out anywhere, anytime, without needing expensive equipment or a gym membership. Whether you're trying to build strength, improve flexibility, or just get moving after a period of inactivity, calisthenics meets you where you are and grows with you.

This chapter is your guide to understanding the basics of calisthenics, focusing on essential exercises, routines, and common pitfalls to avoid. Let's dive in and discover how this accessible form of exercise can transform your body and mind.

WARMING UP: ESSENTIAL WARM-UP ROUTINES FOR INJURY PREVENTION

BEFORE YOU JUMP INTO YOUR WORKOUT, IT'S IMPORTANT TO SET ASIDE A FEW MINUTES TO WARM UP PROPERLY. WHILE IT MIGHT BE TEMPTING TO SKIP THIS STEP, ESPECIALLY WHEN YOU'RE EAGER TO GET STRAIGHT TO THE MAIN EVENT, A GOOD WARM-UP IS KEY TO MAKING YOUR WORKOUT MORE EFFECTIVE AND REDUCING YOUR RISK OF INJURY. THINK OF IT AS PRIMING YOUR BODY FOR THE MOVEMENTS AHEAD—WAKING UP YOUR MUSCLES, GETTING YOUR JOINTS READY TO MOVE, AND INCREASING YOUR HEART RATE GRADUALLY.

Skipping your warm-up can not only increase your chance of getting hurt but also make your workout feel harder. When your body isn't properly prepped, you might find it tougher to get into the groove of your exercises. So, spending just five to ten minutes warming up can make all the difference.

SIMPLE AND EFFECTIVE WARM-UP ROUTINE

A good warm-up doesn't need to be complicated. In fact, it should be simple and easy to follow so that you can make it a consistent part of your routine. The goal is to get your body moving, your blood pumping and your muscles loosened up. Here's a basic warm-up routine that covers all the bases:

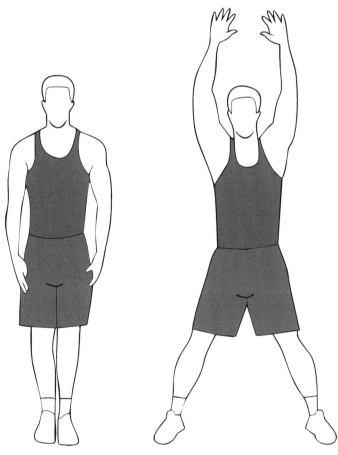

JUMPING JACKS

Jumping jacks are a great way to get your heart rate up quickly. This full-body movement engages your legs, core, and arms, making it an excellent way to kickstart your warm-up.

How to do it: Stand with your feet together and arms at your sides. Jump your feet out to the sides while raising your arms overhead. Jump back to the starting position and repeat.

Duration: Perform jumping jacks for 2-3 minutes to get your blood flowing.

ARM CIRCLES

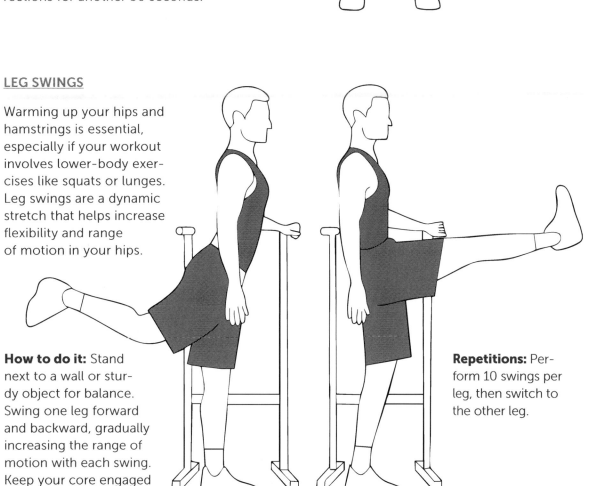

Your shoulders play a significant role in many exercises, especially in calisthenics. Arm circles are a simple way to warm up your shoulder joints and get them ready for action.

How to do it: Stand with your feet shoulder-width apart and extend your arms out to the sides, parallel to the ground. Start making small circles with your arms, gradually increasing the size of the circles.

Duration: Do this for 30 seconds in one direction, then switch directions for another 30 seconds.

LEG SWINGS

Warming up your hips and hamstrings is essential, especially if your workout involves lower-body exercises like squats or lunges. Leg swings are a dynamic stretch that helps increase flexibility and range of motion in your hips.

How to do it: Stand next to a wall or sturdy object for balance. Swing one leg forward and backward, gradually increasing the range of motion with each swing. Keep your core engaged to maintain stability.

Repetitions: Perform 10 swings per leg, then switch to the other leg.

TORSO TWISTS

Your spine and core need to be loose and flexible to handle a wide range of movements during your workout. Torso twists are a simple way to warm up these areas and improve your mobility.

How to do it: Stand with your feet shoulder-width apart and place your hands on your hips. Gently twist your torso to the left, then to the right, making sure to keep your movements controlled.

Duration: Continue twisting for 30 seconds, focusing on loosening up your spine and core muscles.

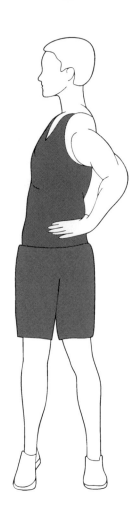

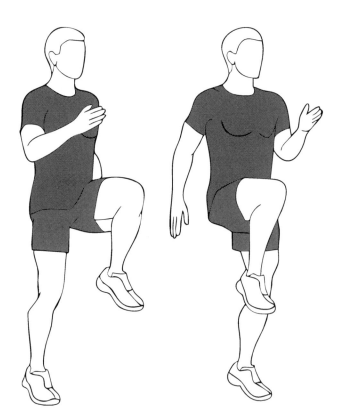

HIGH KNEES

High knees are a dynamic warm-up exercise that gets your heart rate up and engages your core, hip flexors, and legs. This movement is great for loosening up your lower body and preparing it for more intense activities.

How to do it: Stand with your feet hip-width apart and your arms at your sides. Begin jogging in place, lifting your knees as high as possible with each step. Pump your arms as you lift your knees to engage your upper body.

Duration: Perform high knees for 1-2 minutes to elevate your heart rate and warm up your legs and core.

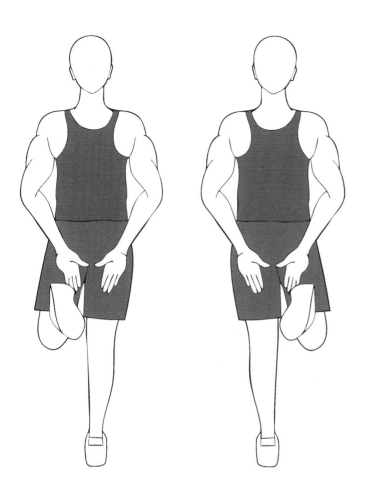

BUTT KICKS

Butt kicks are a simple yet effective warm-up exercise that helps loosen up your quads and improve flexibility in your knees and hips. This movement also increases your heart rate and warms up your lower body.

How to do it: Stand with your feet hip-width apart and your arms at your sides. Begin jogging in place, kicking your heels up toward your glutes with each step. Keep your core engaged and stay light on your feet as you kick your heels back.

Duration: Perform butt kicks for 1-2 minutes to get your heart rate up and warm up your lower body.

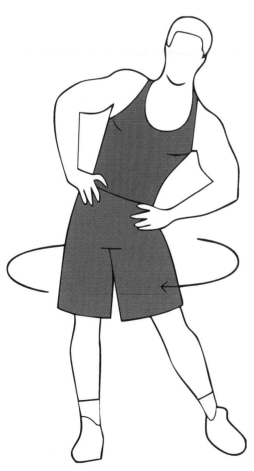

HIP CIRCLES

Hip circles are a great way to warm up your hip joints and improve flexibility in your lower body. This exercise helps loosen up tight hips and prepares you for exercises that involve lower body movement.

How to do it: Stand with your feet shoulder-width apart and place your hands on your hips. Begin making large circles with your hips, rotating them in a smooth motion. Perform 10 circles in one direction, then switch to the opposite direction.

Duration: Do 10-15 hip circles in each direction to loosen up your hips and lower back.

INCHWORM

The inchworm is a dynamic warm-up exercise that stretches your hamstrings, calves, and shoulders while also engaging your core. This movement helps improve flexibility and mobility in your entire body.

How to do it: Stand with your feet hip-width apart and your arms at your sides. Bend forward at your hips and place your hands on the ground in front of you. Slowly walk your hands forward into a plank position. Hold the plank for a moment, then walk your feet toward your hands. Stand up and repeat.

Repetitions: Perform 5-8 inchworms to stretch and warm up your entire body.

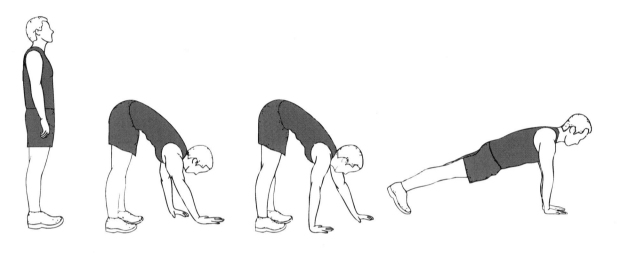

KEEP IT LIGHT AND SIMPLE

Remember, the goal of your warm-up is to get your body ready for exercise, not to wear yourself out. You should feel warm and slightly out of breath by the end of your warm-up, but you shouldn't be fatigued. If you feel tired before your workout even begins, you may have overdone it. Keep things light and easy, focusing on getting your muscles and joints prepped for the movements ahead.

Now that your body is warmed up and ready to go, you can dive into your calisthenics workout with confidence. Whether you're focusing on upper-body strength, lower-body power, or full-body conditioning, a proper warm-up sets the stage for a more effective and safer workout.

FOUNDATIONAL EXERCISES: BUILDING BLOCKS OF CALISTHENICS

IN CALISTHENICS, FOUNDATIONAL EXERCISES FORM THE CORE OF YOUR ROUTINE. THESE EXERCISES RELY ON YOUR BODY WEIGHT TO BUILD STRENGTH, STABILITY, AND ENDURANCE. BY MASTERING THESE MOVES, YOU LAY THE GROUNDWORK FOR MORE ADVANCED CALISTHENICS EXERCISES DOWN THE LINE. BELOW, WE'LL COVER THE KEY EXERCISES EVERY BEGINNER SHOULD FOCUS ON.

PUSH-UPS: VARIATIONS AND PROGRESSIONS

Push-ups are one of the most iconic exercises in calisthenics. They are simple yet powerful for building upper body strength, specifically targeting the chest, shoulders, triceps, and core. Whether you're just beginning your fitness journey or looking to enhance your existing routine, push-ups offer a versatile way to train. What makes them even more appealing is their adaptability. No matter where you are in your fitness journey, there's a push-up variation for you. In this section, we'll explore various push-up progressions that cater to beginner fitness levels. You'll learn how to start with the basics and gradually work your way up to more advanced beginner variations.

STANDARD PUSH-UP

The standard push-up is the foundation of many calisthenics routines. It works multiple muscle groups simultaneously, including the chest, shoulders, triceps, and core. Here's how to perform it:

1. **Start in a plank position:** Place your hands slightly wider than shoulder-width apart. Your feet should be together, and your body should form a straight line from your head to your heels.

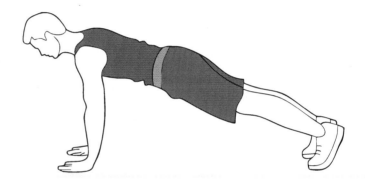

2. **Engage your core:** Make sure your hips don't sag. Engaging your core keeps your body stable and ensures proper alignment.

3. **Lower your body:** Slowly bend your elbows, lowering your chest toward the ground. Keep your elbows at about a 45-degree angle to your torso. Aim to bring your chest as close to the floor as possible without touching it.

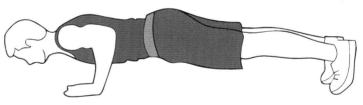

4. **Push back up:** Exhale as you push yourself back up to the starting position, fully extending your arms.

The standard push-up is a challenging exercise for many, especially if you're new to working out. But don't worry—there are several progressions you can follow to build up to the full push-up.

WALL PUSH-UPS

If the standard push-up feels too difficult, wall push-ups are a great starting point. This variation reduces the amount of weight you need to push, making it more manageable for beginners. Wall push-ups are also a good option if you're recovering from an injury and need a gentler way to reintroduce movement.

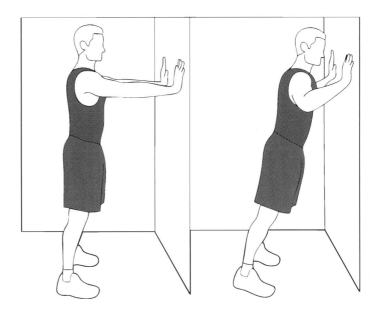

1. **Stand facing a wall:** Position yourself about an arm's length away from the wall. Place your hands on the wall at shoulder height and width.

2. **Engage your core:** Just like with regular push-ups, keeping your core tight helps maintain good form.

3. **Lower your chest:** Bend your elbows and lower your chest toward the wall. Keep your body in a straight line as you do this—no bending at the hips.

4. **Push back:** Exhale as you push yourself back to the starting position.

This variation allows you to focus on form while still building strength. Once you can comfortably perform 15-20 wall push-ups in a row, you're ready to move on to the next progression.

KNEE PUSH-UPS

Knee push-ups are a great intermediary step between wall push-ups and standard push-ups. This variation reduces the intensity by allowing you to rest your knees on the ground, which means you're lifting less of your body weight.

1. **Get into a high plank position:** Start with your hands on the ground, slightly wider than shoulder-width apart. Rest your knees on the floor, creating a straight line from your head to your knees.

2. **Engage your core:** Keeping your core tight prevents your hips from sagging or arching.

3. **Lower your chest:** Slowly bend your elbows and lower your chest toward the ground. Your elbows should stay at a 45-degree angle to your body.

4. **Push back up:** Exhale as you push yourself back to the starting position.

Knee push-ups are a crucial step in your progression. They allow you to build strength in your upper body while still practicing proper push-up form. As you get stronger, you'll feel more confident moving on to the full push-up.

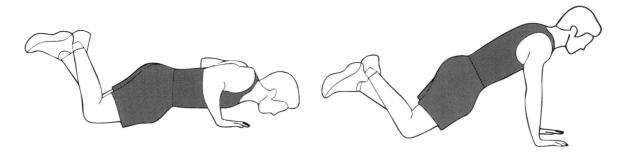

INCLINE PUSH-UPS

Incline push-ups are another excellent way to bridge the gap between knee push-ups and standard push-ups. By elevating your hands on a surface like a bench, chair, or step, you reduce the load on your upper body, making the exercise easier than a standard push-up but more challenging than knee push-ups.

1. **Find an elevated surface:** Place your hands on a stable, elevated surface. The higher the surface, the easier the exercise.

2. **Get into a plank position:** Your body should form a straight line from your head to your heels, just like in a standard push-up.

3. **Lower your chest:** Bend your elbows and lower your chest toward the elevated surface. Keep your elbows at a 45-degree angle to your body.

4. **Push back up:** Exhale as you push yourself back to the starting position.

Incline push-ups are great because you can adjust the difficulty by choosing different heights. As you get stronger, lower the incline until you're ready for standard push-ups.

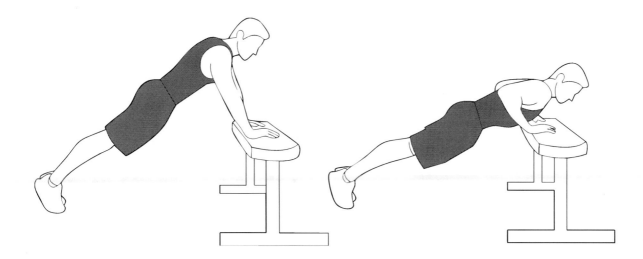

PROGRESSION TIPS

EACH VARIATION BUILDS ON THE LAST, SO PROGRESS AT YOUR OWN PACE. MASTERING ONE LEVEL BEFORE MOVING TO THE NEXT WILL HELP YOU BUILD THE STRENGTH AND CONFIDENCE NEEDED TO KEEP ADVANCING. REMEMBER TO LISTEN TO YOUR BODY AND FOCUS ON MAINTAINING GOOD FORM THROUGHOUT EACH EXERCISE.

SQUATS: BODYWEIGHT AND ASSISTED VARIATIONS

Squats are one of the most fundamental exercises for building lower body strength. They target key muscle groups like your quads, glutes, and hamstrings while also engaging your core. Whether you're new to fitness or experienced in strength training, incorporating squats into your routine can help improve your balance, stability, and overall power. In this section, we'll explore both assisted and bodyweight squats, starting from the basics and progressing as you build confidence and strength.

ASSISTED SQUATS

If you're new to squats or find it challenging to maintain balance, assisted squats are a great starting point. This variation allows you to practice the movement with added stability, reducing the risk of falling or losing your balance. Assisted squats are also helpful if you're recovering from an injury or have limited mobility.

1. **Stand in front of a chair or bench:** Position yourself in front of a sturdy chair, bench, or any other stable object. The chair should be directly behind you so you can use it as a reference point for how low to squat.

2. **Position your feet:** Stand with your feet shoulder-width apart and your toes slightly pointed out. This stance helps you maintain stability as you squat.

3. **Engage your core:** Tighten your core muscles to support your back and maintain good posture throughout the movement.

4. **Sit back:** Begin the squat by pushing your hips back as if you're going to sit in the chair. Bend your knees and lower your body, keeping your chest up and your back straight.

5. **Stop before sitting:** Lower yourself until your thighs are parallel to the ground or just before your butt touches the seat. If you need extra support, you can lightly touch the chair with your hands.

6. **Push through your heels:** Press through your heels and engage your glutes as you stand back up to the starting position.

Assisted squats are an excellent way to build confidence and master the squat form. Once you feel comfortable with the movement and can perform it with ease, you're ready to progress to bodyweight squats.

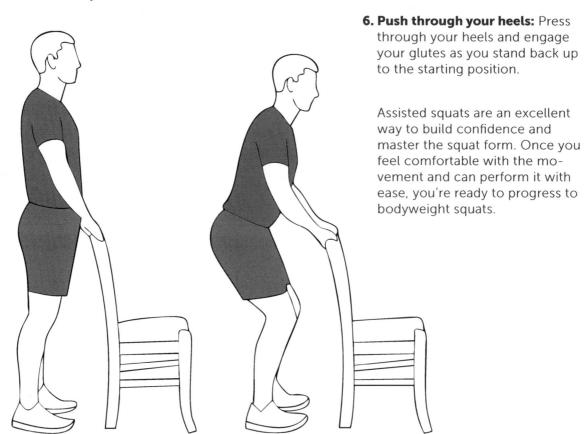

BODYWEIGHT SQUATS

Bodyweight squats are the next step in your squat progression. By removing the assistance of a chair or bench, you'll engage more muscles, particularly in your core, to stabilize your body. This variation requires a bit more strength and control but offers even greater benefits for your lower body.

1. **Stand with your feet shoulder-width apart:** Your feet should be parallel, with your toes slightly turned out. This stance helps you distribute your weight evenly.

2. **Engage your core:** Keep your core muscles tight to support your spine and prevent any excessive arching of your lower back.

3. **Lower your body:** Start the movement by bending your knees and pushing your hips back as if you're sitting in an invisible chair. Keep your chest lifted and your gaze forward.

4. **Check your knee alignment:** Make sure your knees track over your toes, but don't let them extend past your toes. This protects your knees from unnecessary strain.

5. **Go as low as comfortable:** Lower your body until your thighs are parallel to the ground or as far as you can go while maintaining good form. Everyone's range of motion is different, so listen to your body.

6. **Push through your heels:** Drive through your heels to stand back up. Squeeze your glutes at the top of the movement for added activation.

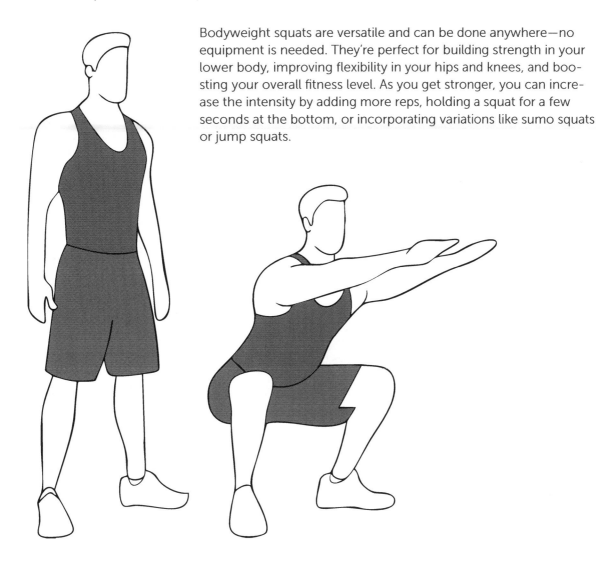

Bodyweight squats are versatile and can be done anywhere—no equipment is needed. They're perfect for building strength in your lower body, improving flexibility in your hips and knees, and boosting your overall fitness level. As you get stronger, you can increase the intensity by adding more reps, holding a squat for a few seconds at the bottom, or incorporating variations like sumo squats or jump squats.

THE NEW CALISTHENICS FORMULA

PLANKS: CORE FOUNDATION

Planks are a foundational exercise in calisthenics and strength training, renowned for their ability to build core strength. Unlike crunches, which primarily target your abdominal muscles, planks engage your entire core, including your lower back, obliques, and glutes. This full-body engagement makes planks a highly effective exercise for improving overall stability, endurance, and strength. Whether you're a beginner or an experienced athlete, planks can be adapted to suit your fitness level and provide a solid base for a stronger core.

FOREARM PLANK

The forearm plank is the most common variation and a great starting point for building core strength. This exercise may look simple, but holding the correct form can be challenging, especially for beginners. It's important to focus on proper alignment to maximize the benefits and avoid strain on your lower back.

1. **Start on your hands and knees:** Position yourself on the floor on all fours. Your hands should be directly under your shoulders, and your knees should be hip-width apart.

2. **Lower onto your forearms:** Drop down onto your forearms so that your elbows are directly under your shoulders. Your forearms should be parallel to each other, with your palms facing down.

3. **Step your feet back:** Extend your legs behind you, one at a time, so that your body forms a straight line from your head to your heels. Your feet should be hip-width apart.

4. **Engage your core:** Tighten your core muscles as if you're bracing for a punch. This helps protect your lower back and keeps your body stable.

5. **Hold the position:** Keep your body in a straight line, avoiding the common mistakes of letting your hips sag or lifting your butt too high. Hold this position for as long as you can while maintaining proper form.

The forearm plank is excellent for building foundational core strength. Start by holding the position for 20-30 seconds and gradually work your way up to longer holds as your strength improves.

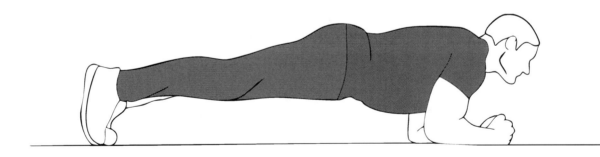

HIGH PLANK

Once you feel comfortable with the forearm plank, you can progress to the high plank. This variation involves holding the plank position on your hands instead of your forearms. The high plank adds an extra challenge to your upper body, particularly your shoulders and arms, while still engaging your core muscles.

1. **Start in a push-up position:** Begin by placing your hands on the floor directly under your shoulders. Your fingers should be spread wide for stability.

2. **Step your feet back:** Extend your legs behind you, one at a time, so your body forms a straight line from your head to your heels. Your feet should be about hip-width apart.

3. **Engage your core:** Tighten your core muscles to prevent your hips from sagging or your lower back from arching. Keep your gaze slightly ahead of you to maintain a neutral neck position.

4. **Hold the position:** Just like in the forearm plank, focus on maintaining a straight line from head to heels. Avoid locking your elbows or letting your shoulders creep up toward your ears.

Planks are an excellent core exercise that provides a strong foundation for many other movements in calisthenics and strength training. Whether you're doing forearm planks or high planks, focus on maintaining proper form and gradually increasing your hold times to build endurance and strength. With consistent practice, you'll notice improvements in your core stability, posture, and overall fitness.

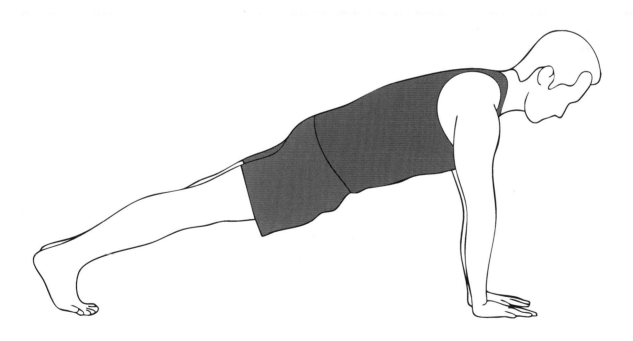

LUNGES: BALANCE AND STRENGTH

Lunges are a fundamental lower body exercise that not only strengthens your legs but also enhances your balance, coordination, and core stability. This movement engages several major muscle groups, including your quads, glutes, and hamstrings. What sets lunges apart from other exercises is their focus on unilateral strength, which means they work one leg at a time. This helps correct muscle imbalances, improve functional movement, and prevent injuries.

Lunges are versatile and can be modified to suit different fitness levels. Whether you're just starting out or looking to take your lower body strength to the next level, lunges should be a staple in your workout routine.

ASSISTED LUNGES

If you're new to lunges or struggle with balance, assisted lunges are a great way to get started. This variation allows you to practice the movement while holding onto a sturdy object for support, reducing the risk of falling or losing your balance.

1. **Stand near a wall or sturdy object:** Position yourself next to a wall, chair, or any stable surface you can hold onto for balance.

2. **Step one foot forward:** Take a big step forward with one foot, creating a split stance. Your front foot should be flat on the ground, and your back foot should be on the ball of your foot.

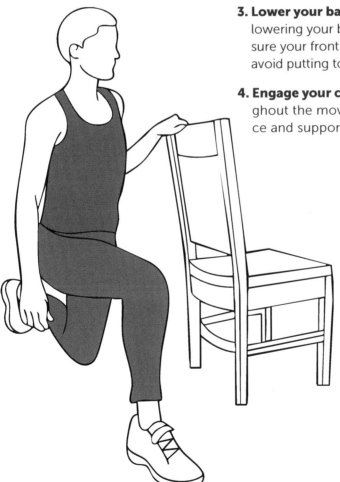

3. **Lower your back knee:** Slowly bend both knees, lowering your back knee toward the ground. Make sure your front knee stays directly over your ankle to avoid putting too much pressure on your knee joint.

4. **Engage your core:** Keep your core tight throughout the movement to help maintain your balance and support your lower back.

5. **Push through your front heel:** Drive through the heel of your front foot to stand back up, returning to the starting position. Use the wall or chair for support as needed.

Assisted lunges are an excellent way to practice proper form and build strength in your legs without worrying about losing your balance. Once you feel confident with this variation, you can progress to bodyweight lunges.

BODYWEIGHT LUNGES

Bodyweight lunges are the next progression after assisted lunges. Without the support of a wall or chair, you'll rely on your core and leg strength to stay balanced throughout the movement. This variation challenges your stability even more, making it an effective exercise for improving coordination and control.

1. **Stand with your feet hip-width apart:** Start in an upright position with your feet about hip-width apart and your hands on your hips or by your sides.

2. **Step forward into a lunge:** Take a big step forward with one foot, creating a split stance. Your front foot should be flat on the ground, and your back foot should be on the ball of your foot.

3. **Lower your back knee:** Bend both knees and lower your back knee toward the ground. Your front knee should be in line with your ankle, and your back knee should hover just above the floor.

4. **Engage your core:** Keep your core muscles engaged to help you maintain balance and stability.

5. **Push through your front heel:** Press through the heel of your front foot to stand back up and return to the starting position.

Lunges are a versatile and effective exercise that can help you build strength, improve balance, and enhance your overall fitness. Whether you're starting with assisted lunges or progressing to bodyweight variations, focus on mastering the technique and gradually increasing the intensity. With consistency, you'll notice significant improvements in your lower body strength and stability, both in your workouts and your daily activities.

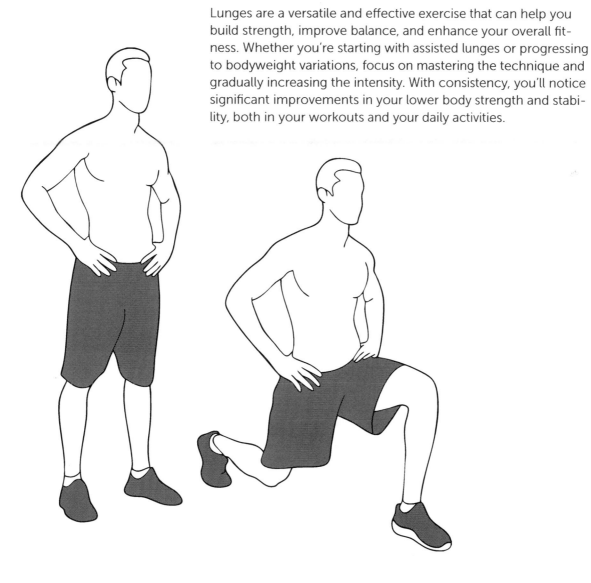

GLUTE BRIDGES: HIP AND CORE ACTIVATION

Glute bridges are a powerful yet simple exercise that targets your glutes and hamstrings while engaging your core. This exercise is particularly beneficial if you spend a lot of time sitting, as it helps to counteract the negative effects of prolonged sitting on your hips and lower back. Glute bridges not only strengthen your lower body but also improve hip mobility and core stability, making them a valuable addition to any fitness routine.

Whether you're looking to build a stronger lower body or improve your posture and flexibility, glute bridges can help you achieve those goals. The best part? You don't need any equipment—just a bit of floor space.

STANDARD GLUTE BRIDGE

The standard glute bridge is a foundational movement that focuses on activating your glutes and hamstrings. It's a simple exercise that can be done anywhere, making it perfect for beginners and advanced exercisers alike.

1. **Lie on your back:** Start by lying flat on your back with your knees bent and your feet flat on the ground. Position your feet hip-width apart, and place your arms at your sides with your palms facing down.

2. **Engage your core:** Before lifting your hips, engage your core muscles by drawing your belly button toward your spine. This will help stabilize your pelvis and protect your lower back during the movement.

3. **Press through your heels:** Push through your heels to lift your hips off the ground. As you lift, squeeze your glutes and create a straight line from your shoulders to your knees.

4. **Hold at the top:** Hold the position for a second or two at the top, focusing on squeezing your glutes and keeping your core engaged.

5. **Lower slowly:** Slowly lower your hips back down to the ground, maintaining control throughout the movement.

The standard glute bridge is a great exercise for activating your glutes and building strength in your hamstrings. Start with 12-15 repetitions, and gradually increase the number of reps as you get stronger.

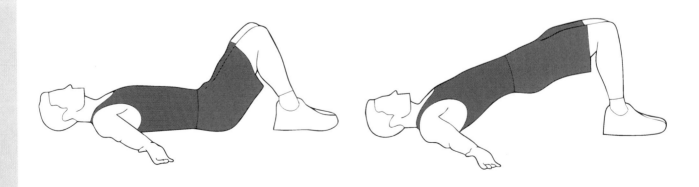

SINGLE-LEG GLUTE BRIDGE

Once you've mastered the standard glute bridge, you can progress to the single-leg glute bridge for an extra challenge. This variation increases the intensity by isolating one leg at a time, which places more demand on your glutes and further engages your core for stability.

1. Lie on your back: Start in the same position as the standard glute bridge, lying on your back with your knees bent and your feet flat on the ground.

2. Extend one leg: Extend one leg straight out, keeping the other foot flat on the ground. Your extended leg should be in line with your torso.

3. Engage your core: As with the standard bridge, engage your core muscles to stabilize your pelvis.

4. Lift your hips: Press through the heel of your grounded foot to lift your hips off the ground. As you lift, squeeze your glutes and maintain a straight line from your shoulders to your knees.

5. Hold and lower: Hold the position at the top for a second or two, then slowly lower your hips back down. Make sure to keep your extended leg straight throughout the movement.

6. Switch sides: After completing the desired number of reps on one side, switch legs and repeat on the other side.

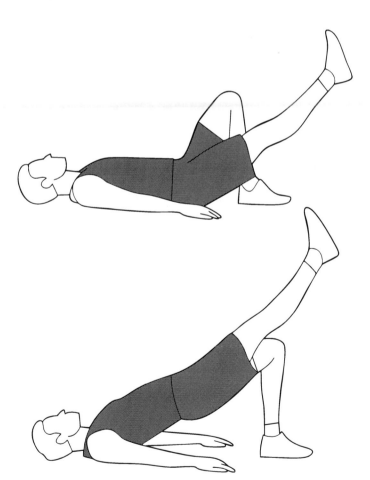

Glute bridges are a versatile and effective exercise that can help you build strength, improve hip mobility, and enhance your overall core stability. Whether you're just starting with the standard glute bridge or progressing to more advanced variations like the single-leg bridge, focus on maintaining proper form and gradually increasing the intensity of your workouts. With consistency, you'll notice significant improvements in your lower body strength and flexibility, both in your workouts and your daily activities.

ASSISTED PULL-UPS AND DIPS

Pull-ups and dips are among the most effective exercises for building upper body strength, targeting your back, shoulders, chest, and arms. However, they can be quite challenging, especially for beginners or those returning to strength training. That's where assisted variations come in handy. By using assistance, you can work through the full range of motion, gradually build strength, and progress toward unassisted pull-ups and dips. These exercises lay the foundation for more advanced calisthenics movements like muscle-ups and handstands.

ASSISTED PULL-UPS

Pull-ups are one of the best exercises for building upper back and biceps strength. They primarily target your lats, but they also engage your shoulders, core, and even your grip. For beginners, assisted pull-ups are a great way to start developing the strength needed to perform full pull-ups unassisted.

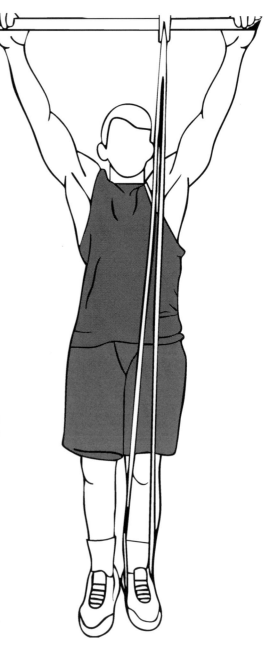

1. **Choose Your Assistance Method:** There are a few ways to assist your pull-ups, including using resistance bands or an assisted pull-up machine at the gym. Resistance bands can be looped over the pull-up bar and stretched under your feet or knees to provide support. Alternatively, the assisted pull-up machine uses counterweights to reduce the amount of weight you're lifting.

2. **Grip the Bar:** Grab the pull-up bar with an overhand grip, slightly wider than shoulder-width apart. Engage your core and keep your body in a straight line.

3. **Engage Your Back Muscles:** As you pull yourself up, focus on engaging your back muscles rather than just relying on your arms. Think about pulling your chest toward the bar, not just lifting your chin over it.

4. **Pull Up:** Use the assistance to help lift your body toward the bar, keeping your core tight and your movements controlled. Avoid swinging or using momentum to complete the movement.

5. **Lower Slowly:** Lower yourself back down with control, focusing on maintaining tension in your muscles throughout the movement.

Assisted pull-ups are a great way to gradually build the strength needed for unassisted pull-ups. Start with a level of assistance that allows you to perform 8-10 reps with good form, and over time, reduce the amount of assistance as you get stronger.

ASSISTED DIPS

Dips are an excellent exercise for developing strength in your triceps, chest, and shoulders. They're also a fundamental movement for more advanced calisthenics exercises, such as muscle-ups. However, dips can be tough to perform, especially if you're just starting out. Assisted dips allow you to practice the movement and build strength without overstraining your muscles.

1. **Start with a Bench or Chair:** For beginners, using a bench or chair is a good starting point. Sit on the edge of the bench with your hands placed on either side of your hips. Your fingers should be gripping the edge, and your feet should be flat on the ground in front of you.

2. **Position Your Feet:** Slide your hips off the bench and walk your feet forward so that your legs are straight or bent slightly. The closer your feet are to your body, the easier the movement will be.

3. **Lower Your Body:** Bend your elbows and lower your body toward the ground, keeping your back close to the bench. Your elbows should point straight back, not flaring out to the sides.

4. **Push Back Up:** Push through your palms to straighten your arms and return to the starting position. Focus on engaging your triceps and chest as you push up.

5. **Progress to Parallel Bars:** As you get stronger, you can progress to parallel bars or dip stations, where you'll perform the dip with your full body weight. Start with assistance from resistance bands or a dip machine if needed.

Assisted pull-ups and dips are foundational exercises that help you build the strength and technique needed for more advanced movements. By starting with assistance and gradually progressing, you'll develop the upper body strength required to perform these exercises unassisted, setting the stage for a stronger, more capable physique.

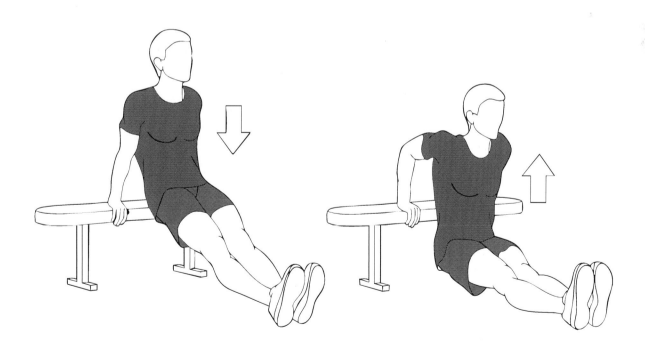

CORE STRENGTHENING EXERCISES FOR BEGINNERS

YOUR CORE IS THE FOUNDATION OF NEARLY EVERY MOVEMENT YOU PERFORM, WHETHER YOU'RE LIFTING WEIGHTS AT THE GYM OR SIMPLY PICKING SOMETHING UP OFF THE FLOOR. A STRONG CORE IMPROVES BALANCE, STABILITY, AND OVERALL STRENGTH WHILE REDUCING YOUR RISK OF INJURY. WHILE PLANKS ARE A FANTASTIC WAY TO BUILD CORE STRENGTH, THERE ARE SEVERAL OTHER BEGINNER-FRIENDLY EXERCISES THAT CAN HELP YOU DEVELOP A WELL-ROUNDED AND FUNCTIONAL CORE. INCORPORATING THESE EXERCISES INTO YOUR ROUTINE WILL NOT ONLY STRENGTHEN YOUR ABS BUT ALSO IMPROVE YOUR ABILITY TO PERFORM EVERYDAY TASKS MORE EFFICIENTLY.

Here are some essential core exercises to get you started:

DEAD BUG

The dead bug is a beginner-friendly exercise that focuses on engaging your deep core muscles, including your transverse abdominis and lower back. This exercise also improves coordination by challenging your ability to move opposing limbs simultaneously while maintaining core stability.

HOW TO DO IT

1. Lie on your back with your arms extended toward the ceiling and your knees bent at a 90-degree angle. Your shins should be parallel to the ground.

2. Engage your core by pressing your lower back into the floor.

3. Slowly lower your right arm and left leg toward the floor, moving them simultaneously. Keep your arm and leg as straight as possible.

4. Stop just before your arm and leg touch the ground, then return to the starting position.

5. Repeat on the opposite side, lowering your left arm and right leg.

Focus on keeping your lower back pressed firmly into the ground throughout the exercise. Avoid letting your back arch as you lower your limbs, as this reduces the effectiveness of the movement. Start with 8-10 repetitions on each side and gradually increase the number as your core gets stronger.

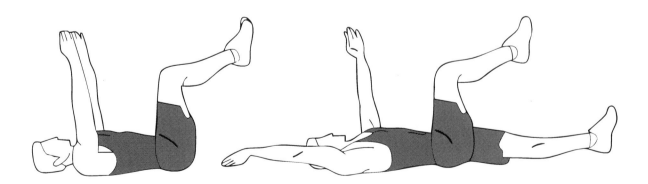

BIRD-DOG

The bird-dog exercise is excellent for building core stability and improving balance. It engages your entire core, including your lower back and glutes, while also challenging your coordination. This movement helps you develop control and stability, which are essential for maintaining proper posture and preventing injury.

HOW TO DO IT

1. Start on your hands and knees in a tabletop position, with your wrists directly under your shoulders and your knees under your hips.
2. Engage your core by pulling your belly button toward your spine.
3. Extend your right arm forward and your left leg back, creating a straight line from your fingertips to your toes.
4. Hold the position for a moment, then slowly return to the starting position.
5. Repeat on the opposite side, extending your left arm and right leg.

Focus on keeping your hips level and your core tight throughout the movement. Avoid letting your lower back arch or your hips twist as you extend your limbs. Start with 8-10 repetitions on each side, holding the extended position for 2-3 seconds, and gradually increase the hold time as you build stability.

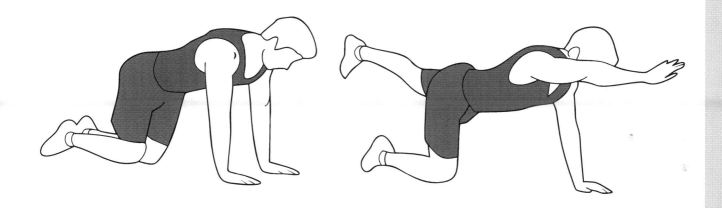

LEG RAISES

Leg raises are a simple yet effective exercise for targeting your lower abs. They help strengthen the muscles that stabilize your pelvis and lower spine, making them a great addition to any core workout routine. This exercise also improves flexibility in your hips and lower back.

HOW TO DO IT

1. Lie on your back with your legs straight and your arms at your sides, palms facing down.
2. Engage your core by pressing your lower back into the ground.
3. Slowly lift your legs toward the ceiling, keeping them as straight as possible. Try to raise them until they form a 90-degree angle with your torso.
4. Lower your legs back down with control, stopping just before they touch the ground.
5. Repeat the movement for the desired number of repetitions.

Keep your core engaged throughout the exercise to prevent your lower back from arching. If you find it difficult to keep your legs straight, you can bend your knees slightly until you build more strength. Start with 8-12 repetitions and gradually increase the number as your lower abs get stronger.

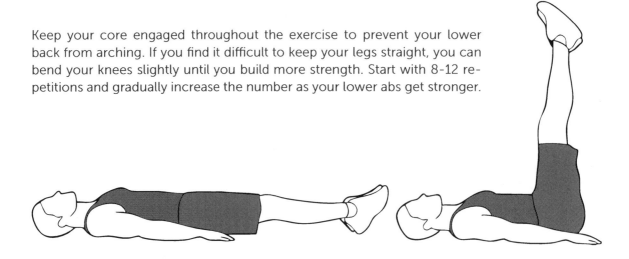

GLUTE BRIDGE MARCH

The glute bridge march combines the benefits of a glute bridge with an added challenge to your core. This exercise targets your glutes, lower back, and core, improving stability and coordination.

HOW TO DO IT

1. Lie on your back with your knees bent and feet flat on the ground, hip-width apart. Place your arms at your sides with palms facing down.
2. Press through your heels to lift your hips off the ground into a glute bridge position, creating a straight line from your shoulders to your knees.
3. While keeping your hips lifted, lift your right foot off the ground and bring your knee toward your chest, then lower it back down.
4. Repeat the movement with your left leg, alternating legs as if you're marching in place.
5. Continue alternating for 8-12 repetitions per leg.

Focus on keeping your hips stable and avoiding any sagging as you march. Engage your core throughout the movement to maintain balance and control.

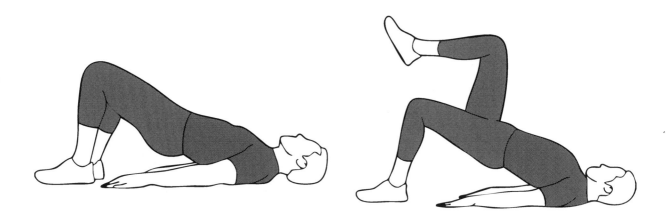

HEEL TAPS

Heel taps are a great exercise for targeting your lower abs and improving core strength. They involve controlled movement, making them a good option for beginners.

HOW TO DO IT

1. Lie on your back with your knees bent and feet flat on the ground. Place your arms at your sides with palms facing down.
2. Lift your legs so that your knees are bent at a 90-degree angle, and your shins are parallel to the ground.
3. Slowly lower your right heel to tap the ground while keeping your lower back pressed into the floor.
4. Bring your right leg back up to the starting position, then lower your left heel to tap the ground.
5. Continue alternating legs for 10-15 repetitions per leg.

Focus on maintaining control throughout the movement and avoid arching your lower back. Keep your core engaged to stabilize your pelvis

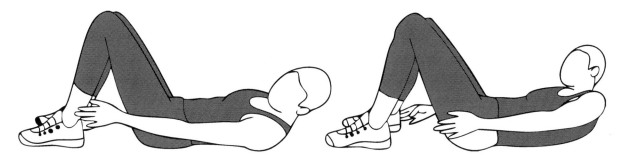

SEATED RUSSIAN TWISTS

Russian twists are an excellent exercise for strengthening your obliques and improving rotational stability. This exercise helps build a strong core and enhances your ability to twist and turn in daily activities.

HOW TO DO IT

1. Sit on the ground with your knees bent and feet flat on the floor. Lean back slightly while keeping your spine straight.
2. Clasp your hands together in front of your chest, or hold a lightweight if you want to increase the challenge.
3. Twist your torso to the right, bringing your hands or the weight toward the floor beside your hip.
4. Return to the center, then twist your torso to the left, bringing your hands or weight toward the floor on the opposite side.
5. Continue alternating sides for 10-12 repetitions per side.

Keep your core tight, and avoid rounding your back as you twist. The movement should come from your core, not just your arms.

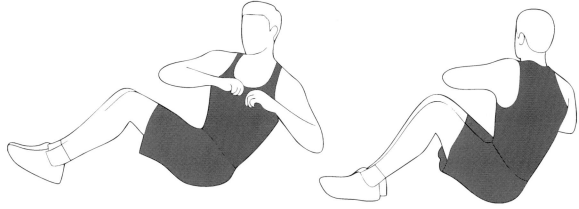

PELVIC TILT

The pelvic tilt is a simple yet effective exercise for engaging your deep core muscles and improving lower back stability. It's particularly helpful for beginners looking to build core strength without putting strain on their back.

HOW TO DO IT

1. Lie on your back with your knees bent and feet flat on the ground. Place your arms at your sides with palms facing down.
2. Engage your core by pressing your lower back into the ground.
3. Tilt your pelvis slightly upward as if you're trying to flatten the curve of your lower back against the floor.
4. Hold the position for a few seconds, then release and relax your pelvis back to its natural position.
5. Repeat the movement for 12-15 repetitions.

Focus on small, controlled movements. The goal is to engage your deep core muscles, so avoid over-arching your back or lifting your hips too high off the floor. By incorporating these beginner-friendly core exercises into your routine, you'll build a strong and stable core that supports your overall fitness and enhances your performance in both workouts and daily activities.

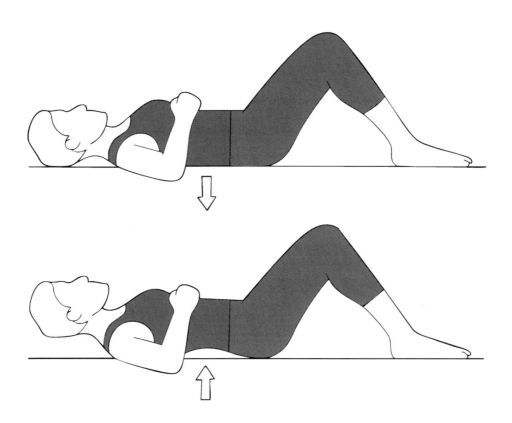

CREATING A ROUTINE: HOW TO STRUCTURE BEGINNER WORKOUTS

NOW THAT YOU'RE FAMILIAR WITH SOME FOUNDATIONAL EXERCISES, IT'S TIME TO CREATE A STRUCTURED WORKOUT ROUTINE. WHEN YOU'RE JUST STARTING OUT, IT'S CRUCIAL TO TAKE THINGS SLOW. YOU WANT TO BUILD A SOLID FOUNDATION WITHOUT OVERWHELMING YOURSELF. STARTING WITH MANAGEABLE WORKOUTS WILL HELP YOU DEVELOP CONSISTENCY, WHICH IS THE KEY TO LONG-TERM PROGRESS. LET'S BREAK DOWN HOW TO STRUCTURE YOUR BEGINNER CALISTHENICS WORKOUTS SO YOU CAN BUILD STRENGTH, IMPROVE YOUR FITNESS, AND STAY MOTIVATED.

WARM-UP

Before you jump into your main workout, warming up is essential. Think of it as preparing your body for what's to come. A good warm-up increases your heart rate, loosens up your muscles, and reduces the risk of injury. For beginners, 5-10 minutes of dynamic stretching and light cardio should do the trick.

- **Jumping Jacks:** Perform jumping jacks for 2-3 minutes to get your heart pumping and your blood flowing.

- **Arm Circles:** Do 30 seconds of arm circles in one direction, then switch and do 30 seconds in the other direction to warm up your shoulders.

- **Leg Swings:** Stand next to a wall or sturdy object for balance and perform 10 leg swings per leg, front to back, to loosen up your hips and hamstrings.

These simple movements help prepare your body for the exercises ahead. Once you're warmed up, it's time to move into the main workout.

MAIN WORKOUT

Your main workout should focus on building strength and endurance using the foundational exercises you've learned. Since you're a beginner, start with 4-6 exercises that target different muscle groups. Perform 3 sets of each exercise, with 8-12 repetitions per set. Take 30-60 seconds of rest between sets to recover. Here's a sample beginner calisthenics workout:

1. **Push-Ups (3 sets of 10 reps):** Push-ups are a fantastic exercise for building upper body strength, targeting your chest, shoulders, triceps, and core.

2. **Bodyweight Squats (3 sets of 12 reps):** Squats are essential for developing lower body strength, especially in your quads, glutes, and hamstrings.

3. **Plank (3 sets of 30 seconds):** Planks help strengthen your core, including your abs, lower back, and glutes.

4. **Lunges (3 sets of 8 reps per leg):** Lunges are great for improving your balance and building strength in your legs and glutes.

5. **Glute Bridges (3 sets of 12 reps):** Glute bridges target your glutes and hamstrings while also activating your core.

Assisted Pull-Ups (3 sets of 8 reps): Pull-ups are challenging, but assisted pull-ups allow you to build the strength needed to eventually perform them unassisted.

This routine covers all major muscle groups, ensuring a balanced workout. You can do this routine 3-4 times per week. As you get stronger, you can increase the number of reps or sets, or try more challenging variations of each exercise.

COOL-DOWN

Just as warming up prepares your body for exercise, cooling down helps bring your body back to a resting state. Cooling down helps prevent muscle soreness and stiffness by gradually reducing your heart rate and stretching your muscles. Spend 5-10 minutes on static stretching to relax your muscles and improve flexibility.

- **Hamstring Stretch:** Sit on the ground with your legs extended in front of you. Reach for your toes while keeping your back straight, and hold the stretch for 20-30 seconds.

- **Quad Stretch:** Stand on one leg, grab your opposite foot, and pull it toward your glutes. Hold the stretch for 20-30 seconds, then switch legs.

- **Shoulder Stretch:** Bring one arm across your chest and use your other hand to gently press your arm toward your body. Hold the stretch for 20-30 seconds on each side.

As a beginner, consistency is key. Start with a routine that feels manageable and gradually increase the intensity as you build strength and confidence. Remember, your journey is about progress, not perfection. Stick with it, and over time, you'll see improvements in your strength, endurance, and overall fitness.

COMMON MISTAKES BEGINNERS MAKE AND HOW TO AVOID THEM

Starting a new exercise routine can be exciting, but avoiding certain pitfalls is key to ensuring steady progress and preventing injury. Here are 10 common mistakes that beginners make and tips on how to avoid them:

1. **Skipping the Warm-Up:** Warming up is crucial for preventing injury. Even if you're short on time, don't skip this step. A proper warm-up prepares your muscles and joints for the work ahead, reducing your risk of strains and sprains. Start with dynamic stretches and light cardio to get your blood flowing.

2. **Poor Form:** Proper form is essential to maximizing the effectiveness of your exercises and avoiding injury. Take your time to learn the correct form for each exercise, and don't rush through your reps. If you're unsure about your form, consider working with a trainer or using a mirror to check your alignment.

3. **Doing Too Much Too Soon:** When motivation is high, it can be tempting to push yourself too hard, too fast. Overdoing it can lead to burnout, injury, or even long-term setbacks. Start with a manageable routine and gradually increase the intensity and volume of your workouts as your strength and endurance improve.

④ **Neglecting Recovery:** Rest and recovery are just as important as the workouts themselves. Overtraining without allowing your body adequate time to recover can lead to fatigue, decreased performance, and injury. Make sure to incorporate rest days into your routine, and listen to your body if you're feeling excessively sore or fatigued.

⑤ **Inconsistent Training:** Consistency is key to making progress in any fitness routine. Skipping workouts or being inconsistent can slow your progress and make it harder to achieve your goals. Set a realistic schedule that you can stick to and make exercise a regular part of your lifestyle.

⑥ **Ignoring Nutrition:** Exercise alone won't lead to optimal results if your diet isn't supporting your efforts. Many beginners overlook the importance of proper nutrition, which is essential for fueling your workouts, aiding recovery, and supporting overall health. Focus on a balanced diet with adequate protein, healthy fats, and carbohydrates to meet your energy needs.

⑦ **Setting Unrealistic Goals:** While it's great to aim high, setting unrealistic goals can lead to frustration and disappointment. If you don't see immediate results, you may feel discouraged and give up. Instead, set achievable short-term goals that keep you motivated and gradually build towards your long-term objectives.

⑧ **Not Staying Hydrated:** Proper hydration is often overlooked by beginners. Staying hydrated before, during, and after your workout is essential for maintaining performance and avoiding fatigue or dizziness. Make it a habit to drink water throughout the day and during your workouts, especially if you're exercising in a hot or humid environment.

⑨ **Focusing Only on One Area:** Many beginners make the mistake of only focusing on one area, like building muscle or losing weight, and neglecting other important aspects of fitness, such as flexibility, mobility, and cardiovascular health. A balanced fitness routine should include strength training, cardio, and flexibility exercises for overall health and wellness.

⑩ **Comparing Yourself to Others:** It's easy to fall into the trap of comparing your progress to others, especially with the prevalence of fitness content on social media. Everyone's fitness journey is different, and comparing yourself to others can lead to unnecessary frustration or self-doubt. Focus on your own progress and celebrate your personal achievements, no matter how small they may seem.

By being mindful of these common mistakes, you'll set yourself up for success in your fitness journey. Start slow, stay consistent, and prioritize both your physical and mental well-being as you work towards your goals.

THE BOTTOM LINE

Calisthenics offers a versatile, accessible way to build strength, improve flexibility, and enhance your overall fitness. By starting with foundational exercises like push-ups, squats, and planks, you'll develop the strength and stability needed to progress to more advanced movements over time. Remember, consistency is key. Stick with your routine, listen to your body, and celebrate your progress along the way. You've got this!

INTERMEDIATE CALISTHENICS WORKOUTS

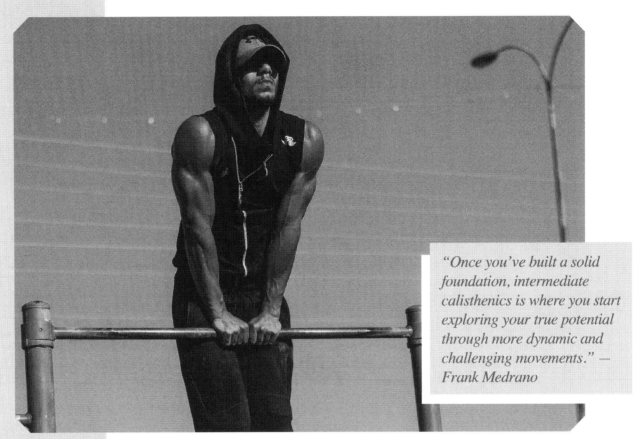

"Once you've built a solid foundation, intermediate calisthenics is where you start exploring your true potential through more dynamic and challenging movements." — Frank Medrano

Congratulations! You've successfully laid the groundwork with your beginner calisthenics routine, and now you're ready to level up. This transition to intermediate calisthenics isn't just about doing more reps or holding a plank longer—it's about refining your form, mastering new techniques, and embracing more challenging movements that will transform your strength, endurance, and overall fitness.

As you move forward, your body will surprise you with its ability to adapt and grow. But with this new level comes a renewed focus on discipline, consistency, and patience. Let's dive into what it takes to advance in your calisthenics journey.

TRANSITIONING TO INTERMEDIATE LEVEL: BUILDING ON YOUR FOUNDATION

YOU'VE MADE IT THIS FAR. THE BASIC CALISTHENICS EXERCISES HAVE SERVED AS YOUR INTRODUCTION TO BODYWEIGHT TRAINING. PUSH-UPS, SQUATS, AND PLANKS HAVE LAID THE GROUNDWORK, STRENGTHENING YOUR MUSCLES, BOOSTING YOUR ENDURANCE, AND IMPROVING YOUR OVERALL BODY AWARENESS. NOW, IT'S TIME TO ELEVATE YOUR TRAINING. TRANSITIONING FROM BEGINNER TO INTERMEDIATE CALISTHENICS IS A CRUCIAL STEP IN YOUR FITNESS JOURNEY. IT'S NOT JUST ABOUT INCREASING THE DIFFICULTY OF YOUR WORKOUTS; IT'S ABOUT REFINING YOUR TECHNIQUE, ENHANCING CONTROL, AND MASTERING BALANCE.

THE IMPORTANCE OF A SOLID FOUNDATION

Before diving into more advanced exercises, take a moment to appreciate the foundation you've built. Think of your body as a structure and the exercises you've been practicing as the foundation of that structure. Without a strong base, the entire system risks collapsing. Push-ups, pull-ups, squats, and planks not only strengthen your muscles but also condition your tendons and ligaments. This conditioning is essential for preventing injuries when you start pushing your body to new limits.

Maintaining good form is crucial. The basics may seem easy now, but this is the perfect time to refine them. If your push-ups are shaky or your squats don't reach full depth, work on correcting these issues before moving on. Quality over quantity is a principle that should guide you through every stage of your fitness journey. Proper form ensures that you target the right muscles and reduce the risk of strain or injury.

WHY TRANSITIONING MATTERS

At the beginner level, your body adapts to the new demands of regular exercise. But by now, those beginner workouts are no longer as challenging as they once were. While consistency is vital, sticking to the same routine can lead to a plateau. Progress is all about pushing your boundaries, and stepping into the intermediate level is where you'll start to see significant changes. This is when your hard work begins to pay off. Your muscles will become more defined, your strength will increase, and your endurance will improve.

Transitioning is also about understanding your body on a deeper level. You've learned the basics, and now you're ready to take on new challenges. But don't rush this process. Sustainable progress is the goal, not quick results. Pay attention to your form, listen to your body, and be patient with yourself. Every small improvement is a step forward.

INCORPORATING ADVANCED MOVEMENTS

Now that you understand the importance of a solid foundation and the need for progression, it's time to explore new exercises. Intermediate calisthenics introduces more complex movements that challenge your control, balance, and strength. Exercises like dips, pistol squats, and archer push-ups require not just strength but also coordination and stability. These movements engage multiple muscle groups simultaneously, helping you build functional strength.

Start by incorporating these new exercises gradually. Add one or two intermediate movements to your routine, and focus on mastering them before adding more. Remember, the goal is to enhance your overall performance, not just to complete more reps or lift heavier. Take your time with each movement, paying close attention to your form and technique. This will ensure that you're getting the most out of each exercise while minimizing the risk of injury.

BALANCING WORKOUTS FOR COMPREHENSIVE STRENGTH

As you transition to intermediate calisthenics, balancing your workouts becomes more important. It's not just about pushing your limits; it's about creating a well-rounded routine that targets all major muscle groups. This means combining pushing exercises like push-ups and dips with pulling exercises like pull-ups and rows. Don't neglect your lower body either—pistol squats and lunges will ensure your legs get the attention they need.

Incorporating core exercises is also crucial. A strong core is the foundation of almost every movement in calisthenics, providing stability and balance. Movements like hanging leg raises, planks with variations, and hollow body holds will strengthen your core, improving your overall performance.

LISTEN TO YOUR BODY

As you take on more advanced exercises, listening to your body becomes even more important. Pushing yourself is necessary for progress, but overtraining can lead to injuries that set you back. Pay attention to how your body feels during and after workouts. If you experience pain, especially in your joints, take a step back and reassess your form or intensity. Rest days are just as important as workout days; they allow your muscles to recover and grow stronger.

CELEBRATING SMALL WINS

Transitioning to intermediate calisthenics is a significant achievement. Celebrate your progress, no matter how small it may seem. Whether it's mastering a new movement, increasing your reps, or simply feeling stronger, these are all signs that you're on the right track. Remember, this journey is about progress, not perfection.

INTERMEDIATE EXERCISES TO TARGET THE WHOLE BODY

NOW THAT YOU'RE READY TO CHALLENGE YOURSELF, LET'S INTRODUCE SOME INTERMEDIATE EXERCISES. THESE MOVES WILL ENGAGE MORE MUSCLE GROUPS, REQUIRE GREATER COORDINATION, AND PUSH YOUR BODY IN NEW WAYS. BY INCORPORATING THEM INTO YOUR ROUTINE, YOU'LL DEVELOP FUNCTIONAL STRENGTH THAT BENEFITS YOU IN DAILY LIFE AS WELL AS IN YOUR CALISTHENICS JOURNEY.

PUSH-UPS: DIAMOND AND ARCHER VARIATIONS

Push-ups are a cornerstone of calisthenics, and by now, you've probably mastered the standard version. Ready to level up? Diamond and archer push-ups are excellent progressions that demand more strength, stability, and control. These variations not only challenge your muscles differently but also help break through plateaus and build balanced upper body strength.

DIAMOND PUSH-UPS

Diamond push-ups take the basic push-up and focus the effort on your triceps and shoulders, providing a unique challenge that also engages your chest and core. Here's how to do them:

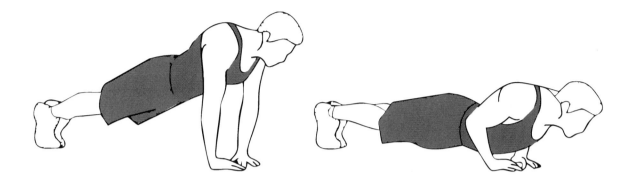

1. **Start in a standard push-up position:** Begin by positioning yourself in the traditional push-up stance with your hands shoulder-width apart, your body in a straight line from head to heels, and your core engaged.

2. **Form the diamond shape with your hands:** Bring your hands together beneath your chest, with your thumbs and index fingers touching to form a diamond or triangle shape. This hand placement shifts the emphasis to your triceps.

3. **Lower your body:** Keep your elbows close to your body, and lower yourself down slowly until your chest is just above your hands. Focus on maintaining a straight line from your head to your heels, and engage your core to prevent sagging.

4. **Push back up:** Press through your hands, straightening your arms to return to the starting position. Squeeze your triceps at the top of the movement for maximum effect.

5. **Repeat:** Aim for 10-12 repetitions per set, ensuring that each rep is controlled and your form is solid. Quality is more important than quantity.

ARCHER PUSH-UPS

Archer push-ups are a significant step up from standard push-ups, providing an intense workout that focuses on unilateral strength—meaning it works one side of your body at a time. This variation not only builds strength but also improves balance and coordination.

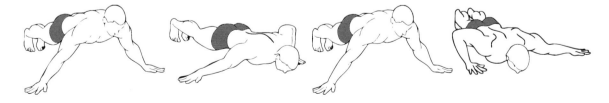

1. **Start in a wide push-up position:** Begin in a push-up stance, but place your hands wider than shoulder-width apart. Your body should still form a straight line from head to heels.

2. **Lower to one side:** As you lower yourself, bend one elbow and keep the opposite arm straight, guiding your body weight toward the bent arm. Imagine you're pulling back a bow-string, hence the name "Archer."

3. **Engage your core:** Keep your core tight to maintain stability. Your straight arm should remain engaged, acting as a guide while your bent arm does most of the work.

4. **Push back up:** Press through the hand of the bent arm to push yourself back to the starting position, ensuring you maintain control throughout the movement.

5. **Alternate sides:** Repeat the movement, this time bending the opposite arm. Aim for 8-10 reps on each side, maintaining good form.

Diamond and archer push-ups are excellent exercises for transitioning from beginner to intermediate calisthenics. They challenge your muscles in new ways, helping you build strength, stability, and control. As you progress, remember to focus on form, gradually increase the difficulty, and listen to your body. These variations will not only make your upper body stronger but will also prepare you for even more advanced calisthenics movements down the road.

PULL-UPS AND CHIN-UPS: MASTERING FULL-RANGE MOVEMENTS

Transitioning from assisted pull-ups or chin-ups to full-range versions is a significant milestone in your calisthenics journey. These exercises are some of the most effective for building upper body strength, as they require you to lift your entire body weight using just your arms and back. Mastering pull-ups and chin-ups not only improves your physical strength but also boosts your confidence as you tackle more challenging movements.

PULL-UPS

Pull-ups are the ultimate test of upper body strength. They primarily target your lats (latissimus dorsi), which are the large muscles on either side of your back. Pull-ups also work your biceps, shoulders, and core, making them a comprehensive upper-body exercise.

1. **Start with an overhand grip:** Grasp the pull-up bar with your palms facing away from you, hands slightly wider than shoulder-width apart.

2. **Engage your core:** Before you start the movement, engage your core muscles to stabilize your body. This will help prevent swinging and ensure that you're using your upper body muscles effectively.

3. **Pull yourself up:** Using your lats and biceps, pull your body upwards until your chin is above the bar. Focus on leading the movement with your chest rather than just pulling with your arms.

4. Pause at the top: Once your chin is above the bar, pause for a moment to fully engage the muscles. This brief pause helps build strength and control.

5. Lower yourself down slowly: Control the descent by lowering yourself back down in a slow and controlled manner until your arms are fully extended. This is the negative phase of the pull-up, which is just as important as the upward movement.

6. Repeat: Aim for 5-8 repetitions per set, focusing on maintaining good form throughout each rep. Quality over quantity is key.

CHIN-UPS

Chin-ups are similar to pull-ups but with an underhand grip. This variation places more emphasis on your biceps while still working your lats and shoulders. Chin-ups are often considered slightly easier than pull-ups, making them a great starting point for those transitioning from assisted to full-range movements.

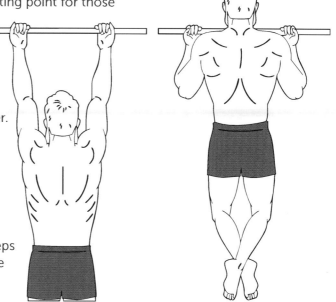

1. Start with an underhand grip: Grasp the pull-up bar with your palms facing towards you, hands shoulder-width apart or slightly closer.

2. Engage your core: Just like with pull-ups, engage your core to stabilize your body and prevent swinging.

3. Pull yourself up: Pull your body upwards, focusing on using your biceps and lats. Aim to bring your chin above the bar, keeping your elbows close to your body.

4. Pause at the top: Once your chin is above the bar, pause briefly to maximize muscle engagement.

5. Lower yourself down slowly: Lower yourself back down in a controlled manner until your arms are fully extended. The slower you go, the more you'll build strength in your muscles.

6. Repeat: Aim for 5-8 repetitions per set, ensuring each rep is performed with proper form.

Mastering full-range pull-ups and chin-ups is a significant achievement in calisthenics. These exercises are a true test of upper body strength and provide immense benefits for your lats, biceps, shoulders, and core. By focusing on controlled movements and full range of motion, you'll build the strength and endurance needed to progress to even more advanced calisthenics movements. Stay consistent, listen to your body, and enjoy the progress you make with each rep.

DIPS: PARALLEL BAR DIPS AND BENCH DIPS

Dips are a cornerstone exercise in calisthenics, especially for developing upper body strength. They effectively target your chest, shoulders, and triceps, making them an essential part of any intermediate workout routine. As you advance, incorporating both parallel bar dips and bench dips will help you build the pushing power necessary for more complex movements.

PARALLEL BAR DIPS

Parallel bar dips are a more advanced variation that requires you to lift and lower your entire body weight.
This exercise primarily targets your triceps, but it also engages your chest, shoulders, and core.

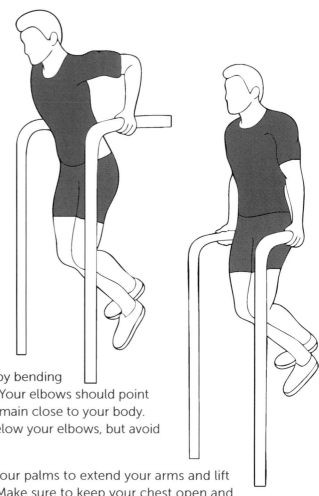

1. **Start with the setup:** Find a set of parallel bars that are shoulder-width apart. Grip the bars firmly with your palms facing inward, and lift yourself up so that your arms are fully extended and your body is straight.

2. **Engage your core**: Before you start the movement, engage your core muscles to stabilize your body. Keep your legs together and slightly bent at the knees.

3. **Lower your body:** Slowly lower yourself by bending your elbows and leaning slightly forward. Your elbows should point backward, and your upper arms should remain close to your body. Lower yourself until your shoulders are below your elbows, but avoid going too low to prevent shoulder strain.

4. **Push yourself back up:** Press through your palms to extend your arms and lift your body back to the starting position. Make sure to keep your chest open and your shoulders down, away from your ears.

5. **Repeat**: Aim for 8-10 repetitions per set, focusing on maintaining proper form throughout the movement. Quality reps are more important than quantity.

BENCH DIPS

Bench dips are a slightly easier variation that focuses more on your triceps. They're a great starting point if you're building up the strength needed for parallel bar dips.

1. **Set up with a bench:** Sit on the edge of a sturdy bench or chair and place your hands next to your hips, fingers pointing forward. Extend your legs out in front of you with your heels on the ground.

2. **Slide off the bench:** Shift your hips off the bench so that your body is supported by your arms. Your legs should be straight, and your back should be close to the bench.

3. Lower your body: Bend your elbows and lower your body toward the floor. Keep your elbows pointing straight back and your shoulders down. Lower yourself until your elbows form a 90-degree angle or as far as your mobility allows.

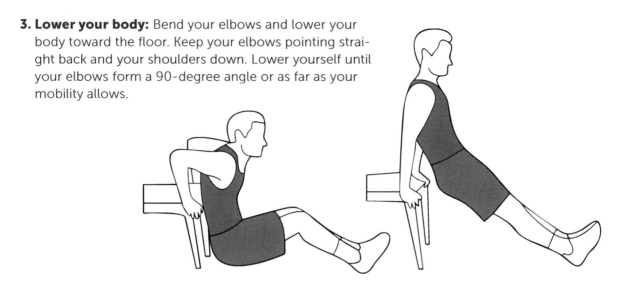

4. Push yourself back up: Press through your palms to straighten your arms and lift your body back to the starting position. Focus on squeezing your triceps at the top of the movement.

5. Repeat: Aim for 10-15 repetitions per set. As you get stronger, you can increase the difficulty by placing your feet on another bench or adding weight to your lap.

Incorporating dips into your calisthenics routine is essential for building upper body strength, particularly in your chest, shoulders, and triceps. Both parallel bar dips and bench dips offer unique benefits, with the former providing a more challenging full-body movement and the latter focusing more on triceps isolation. Start with bench dips to build strength and confidence, and gradually progress to parallel bar dips as you get stronger. By focusing on form, controlled movement, and proper progression, you'll develop the pushing power needed to excel in calisthenics.

PISTOL SQUATS AND JUMP SQUATS

Lower body strength is just as crucial as upper body power when it comes to calisthenics. Strong legs provide the foundation for many movements, from jumping and sprinting to stabilizing your body during more complex exercises. Pistol squats and jump squats are two advanced exercises that challenge your legs, balance, and coordination, pushing your l ower body strength to new levels.

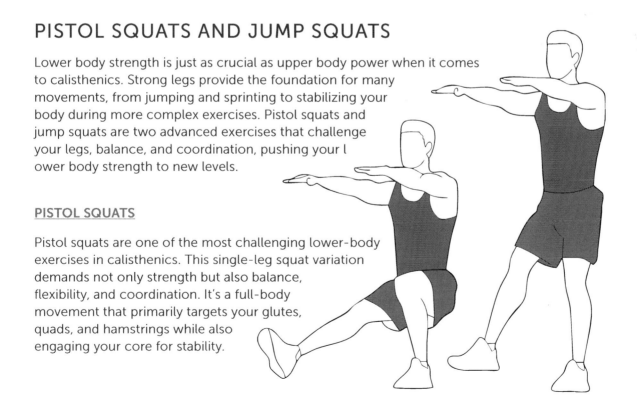

PISTOL SQUATS

Pistol squats are one of the most challenging lower-body exercises in calisthenics. This single-leg squat variation demands not only strength but also balance, flexibility, and coordination. It's a full-body movement that primarily targets your glutes, quads, and hamstrings while also engaging your core for stability.

1. **Start with balance:** Stand on one leg with your other leg extended straight out in front of you. Keep your arms extended forward for balance. This is your starting position.

2. **Lower your body:** Slowly lower yourself into a squat by bending your standing leg while keeping the other leg extended in front of you. Go as low as you can, ideally until your thigh is parallel to the ground or lower. Keep your chest up and your back straight throughout the movement.

3. **Engage your core:** Your core should remain engaged to help maintain balance and prevent your torso from leaning too far forward.

4. **Push through your heel:** Drive through the heel of your standing leg to push yourself back up to the starting position. Focus on using your glutes and quads to power the movement.

5. **Repeat:** Aim for 5-8 repetitions on each leg, ensuring you maintain control and proper form throughout the exercise.

JUMP SQUATS

Jump squats add a plyometric element to your lower body workout, requiring explosive power and endurance. This exercise not only strengthens your legs but also boosts your cardiovascular fitness, making it a great addition to any workout routine.

1. **Start in a squat position:** Stand with your feet shoulder-width apart and lower your body into a squat by bending your knees and pushing your hips back. Keep your chest lifted and your core engaged.

2. **Prepare to jump:** As you reach the bottom of the squat, push through your heels and explode upwards, jumping as high as you can. Swing your arms upward to help generate more power.

3. **Land softly:** As you land, bend your knees to absorb the impact and immediately lower yourself back into the squat position. Your landing should be controlled, with your feet landing softly on the balls of your feet before your heels touch the ground.

4. **Repeat:** Perform 10-15 repetitions, focusing on maintaining explosive power with each jump. Keep your movements controlled and ensure your form remains solid throughout the exercise.

Pistol squats and jump squats are powerful exercises that take your lower body training to the next level. These advanced movements challenge your strength, balance, and coordination, helping you build a more balanced and powerful physique. Start with assisted variations if needed, and gradually progress as you build strength and confidence.

By incorporating these exercises into your routine, you'll enhance your lower body strength, improve your overall athleticism, and achieve a more balanced approach to calisthenics.

HANGING LEG RAISES FOR CORE STRENGTH

Your core plays a crucial role in almost every calisthenics movement. It provides stability, balance, and power, making it essential to develop a strong core if you want to progress in your training. Hanging leg raises are one of the most effective exercises for building core strength. This exercise not only targets your abs but also engages your hip flexors, lower back, and even your grip strength as you hang from a pull-up bar.

HOW TO PERFORM HANGING LEG RAISES

To get the most out of hanging leg raises, it's important to focus on controlled movements and proper form. Here's how to do them:

1. **Start with a proper grip:** Find a sturdy pull-up bar and grip it with your hands shoulder-width apart. Hang with your arms fully extended and your body in a straight line. Your feet should be off the ground, and your core should be engaged to prevent swinging.

2. **Engage your core:** Before you begin the movement, engage your core by tightening your abdominal muscles. This will help stabilize your body and prevent you from using momentum.

3. **Lift your legs:** Slowly lift your legs towards the bar, keeping them as straight as possible. Aim to bring your toes as close to the bar as you can. Focus on using your core muscles to lift your legs rather than relying on momentum.

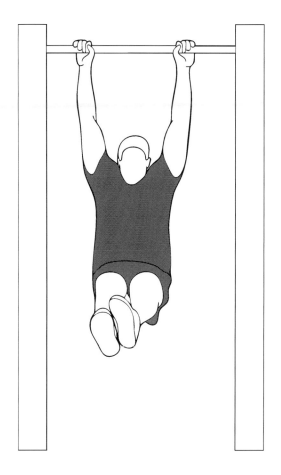

4. **Pause at the top:** Once your legs are fully raised, pause for a moment to maximize muscle engagement. This brief hold helps build strength and control.

5. **Lower your legs slowly:** Lower your legs back down in a slow and controlled manner until they return to the starting position. Avoid letting your body swing or using momentum to lower your legs.

6. **Repeat:** Aim for 8-10 repetitions per set, maintaining control and proper form throughout the exercise.

Hanging leg raises are an excellent exercise for building core strength, essential for progressing in calisthenics and improving your overall fitness. By focusing on controlled movements and gradually increasing the difficulty, you can develop a powerful core that supports a wide range of advanced exercises. Start with bent-knee raises if needed, and work your way up to full straight-leg raises as your strength and technique improve. With consistency and proper form, hanging leg raises will help you achieve a strong, stable core that enhances your performance in calisthenics and beyond.

BULGARIAN SPLIT SQUATS: ENHANCING LEG STRENGTH AND STABILITY

Bulgarian split squats are a single-leg exercise that targets your quads, glutes, and hamstrings while also improving your balance and stability. This intermediate exercise is perfect for building lower body strength and muscle symmetry, as it allows you to work each leg independently.

HOW TO PERFORM BULGARIAN SPLIT SQUATS

1. **Set up with a bench:** Stand a couple of feet in front of a bench or step, with your back facing it. Place the top of one foot on the bench behind you.

2. **Position your front leg:** Your front leg should be far enough forward that when you lower yourself, your knee stays over your ankle and does not extend past your toes.

3. **Lower your body:** Slowly bend your front knee to lower your body towards the ground. Keep your torso upright and your core engaged. Lower yourself until your front thigh is parallel to the ground or slightly below.

4. **Push through your heel:** Drive through the heel of your front foot to return to the starting position. Squeeze your glutes at the top of the movement for maximum engagement.

5. **Repeat:** Aim for 8-12 repetitions on each leg, then switch to the other leg. Maintain control and proper form throughout the exercise.

Incorporating Bulgarian split squats into your routine can significantly enhance leg strength, balance, and stability. This versatile exercise corrects muscle imbalances and improves overall athletic performance, making it a must-add to your workout plan. Start with bodyweight to perfect your form, and gradually increase the intensity for continued growth and progress.

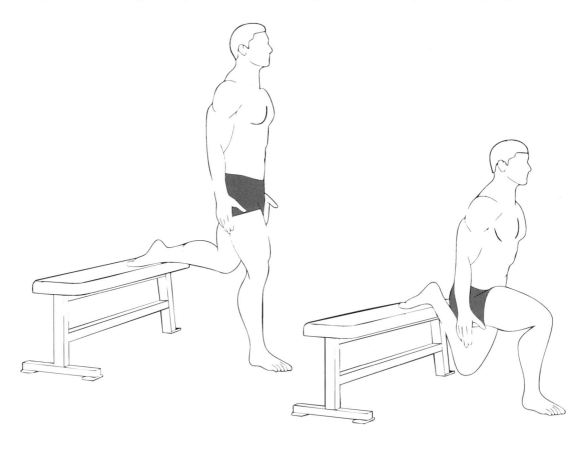

TUCK PLANCHE: STRENGTHENING CORE AND UPPER BODY STABILITY

The tuck planche is an intermediate calisthenics exercise that requires a strong core, shoulders, and triceps. This move involves balancing your body on your hands while keeping your legs tucked, and it's a precursor to the more advanced full planche. The tuck planche not only builds strength but also improves your balance and body control.

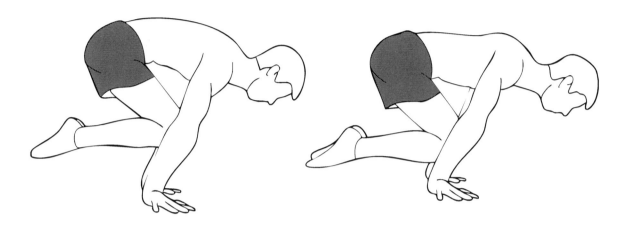

HOW TO PERFORM TUCK PLANCHE

1. Start in a frog stance: Begin by placing your hands on the ground shoulder-width apart. Bend your elbows slightly and place your knees on the outside of your arms, similar to a frog stance in yoga.

2. Lift your feet off the ground: Slowly shift your weight forward onto your hands, engaging your core and lifting your feet off the ground. Keep your knees tucked tightly toward your chest.

3. Engage your shoulders and core: Focus on using your shoulders to stabilize your upper body and your core to keep your hips lifted. Your arms should remain bent slightly to avoid locking out your elbows.

4. Hold the position: Once you've lifted your body off the ground, aim to hold the tuck planche for as long as possible. Start with shorter holds (5-10 seconds) and work up to longer durations.

5. Lower your body: After holding the position, slowly lower your feet back to the ground, maintaining control throughout the movement.

6. Repeat: Aim for 3-5 sets of 5-10 second holds, gradually increasing the hold time as you build strength.

Mastering the tuck planche is a significant step in building upper body and core strength, essential for advancing in calisthenics. By consistently practicing and gradually increasing hold times, you'll enhance your stability, balance, and overall body control. Start with foundational moves like the frog stand, and progress at your own pace to unlock more challenging exercises like the full planche.

ARCHER PULL-UPS:
ENHANCING UNILATERAL BACK AND BICEP STRENGTH

Archer pull-ups are an intermediate calisthenics exercise that targets your back, biceps, and shoulders with an emphasis on unilateral strength. This exercise involves pulling your body up to one side at a time, which not only builds strength but also prepares you for more advanced exercises like one-arm pull-ups.

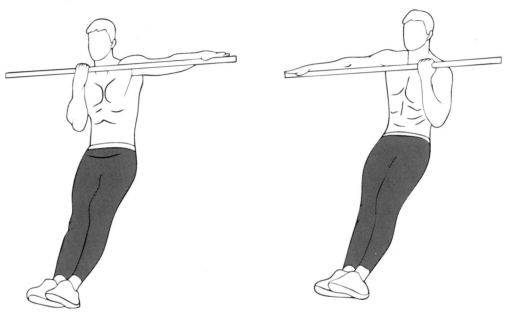

HOW TO PERFORM ARCHER PULL-UPS

1. Start with a wide grip: Find a sturdy pull-up bar and grip it with your hands much wider than shoulder-width apart. Your palms should face away from you (overhand grip).

2. Engage your core: Tighten your core muscles to stabilize your body and prevent swinging during the exercise.

3. Pull yourself up to one side: Begin the pull-up by shifting your weight to one side and pulling your chin towards the hand on that side. Keep the opposite arm straight while pulling with the bent arm.

4. Pause at the top: Once your chin reaches the bar, pause briefly to engage your muscles fully.

5. Lower yourself down slowly: Lower yourself back to the starting position in a controlled manner, ensuring you don't swing.

6. Alternate sides: On the next rep, pull yourself up to the opposite side. Continue alternating sides with each rep.

7. Repeat: Aim for 6-10 repetitions on each side, focusing on control and symmetry in your movement.

Archer pull-ups are a key exercise for building unilateral strength in your back, biceps, and shoulders. By isolating each side, you can correct muscle imbalances and prepare for advanced movements like the one-arm pull-up. Focus on controlled movement and symmetry as you progress, starting with assisted variations if necessary. Incorporating archer pull-ups into your routine will enhance your overall upper-body strength and stability.

TYPEWRITER PUSH-UPS: BUILDING CHEST, SHOULDER, AND TRICEPS STRENGTH

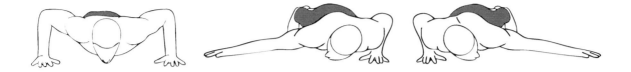

Typewriter push-ups are an intermediate calisthenics exercise that adds a lateral movement component to the traditional push-up. This exercise focuses on building strength in your chest, shoulders, and triceps while also improving your control and stability as you shift your body weight from side to side.

<u>HOW TO PERFORM TYPEWRITER PUSH-UPS</u>

1. Start in a wide push-up position: Get into a standard push-up position but with your hands placed wider than shoulder-width apart. Your feet should also be spread slightly wider for better stability.

2. Lower your body: Begin by lowering yourself into a push-up, but instead of going straight down, shift your weight to one side so that most of your body weight is over one hand. Keep your elbows close to your body.

3. Move laterally: Once you're at the bottom of the push-up on one side, shift your body weight across to the other side, keeping your chest low to the ground. Imagine you're tracing a line from one hand to the other.

4. Push back up: After moving across to the opposite side, push yourself back up to the starting position.

5. Repeat on the other side: Perform the next repetition by lowering yourself and shifting your weight to the opposite side first, then moving across.

6. Repeat: Aim for 6-10 repetitions on each side, focusing on smooth, controlled movements and maintaining proper form.

Typewriter push-ups are an excellent exercise for building upper body strength, control, and stability. By incorporating lateral movement, they challenge your chest, shoulders, triceps, and core in a unique way, making them a valuable addition to your calisthenics routine. Start with foundational push-ups and progress gradually to ensure proper form and maximize the benefits of this dynamic exercise.

INCREASING INTENSITY: INCORPORATING PLYOMETRICS AND TEMPO CHANGES

AFTER MASTERING THE BASICS AND BUILDING A SOLID FOUNDATION WITH INTERMEDIATE CALISTHE-NICS EXERCISES, IT'S TIME TO ELEVATE YOUR WORKOUT ROUTINE. ONE OF THE MOST EFFECTIVE WAYS TO DO THIS IS BY INCORPORATING PLYOMETRICS AND TEMPO CHANGES INTO YOUR EXERCISES. THE-SE TECHNIQUES ARE DESIGNED TO CHALLENGE YOUR MUSCLES IN NEW WAYS, PROMOTING NOT ONLY MUSCLE GROWTH BUT ALSO ENDURANCE AND OVERALL FITNESS. BY ADDING EXPLOSIVE MOVEMENTS AND VARYING THE SPEED OF YOUR EXERCISES, YOU CAN PREVENT YOUR WORKOUTS FROM BECOMING MONOTONOUS WHILE CONTINUOUSLY PUSHING YOUR LIMITS.

PLYOMETRICS: EXPLOSIVE MOVEMENTS FOR POWER

Plyometric exercises are all about generating maximum force in the shortest amount of time. These explosive movements are a fantastic way to develop power, speed, and coordination. When you include plyometrics in your routine, you're not just working on building muscle; you're also enhancing your athletic performance by training your body to move more efficiently and explosively.

BOX JUMPS

Box jumps are a staple in plyometric training. They are simple but highly effective at building explosive power in your legs and improving car-diovascular endurance.

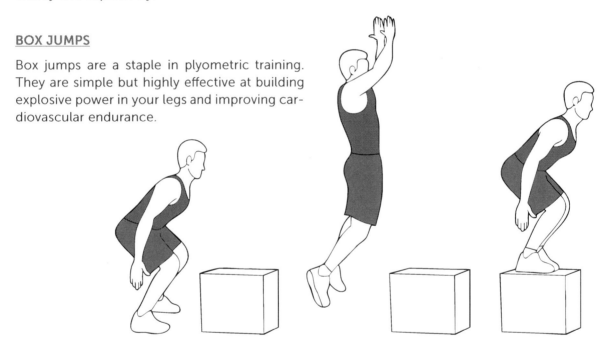

Step 1: Stand in front of a sturdy box or bench, feet shoulder-width apart.
Step 2: Bend your knees slightly, swing your arms back, and explosively jump onto the box.
Step 3: Land softly with both feet on the box, ensuring your knees are slightly bent to absorb the impact.
Step 4: Stand up straight, then step down one foot at a time.
Step 5: Repeat for the desired number of reps.

Box jumps engage your quads, hamstrings, glutes, and calves, making them a comprehensive lower-body exercise. They also get your heart rate up, adding a cardiovascular component to your strength training.

CLAPPING PUSH-UPS

Clapping push-ups take the traditional push-up to the next level by adding an explosive element that targets your upper body power.

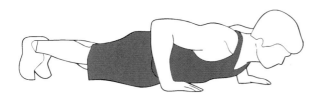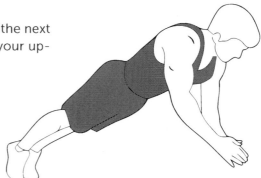

Step 1: Start in a standard push-up position with your hands slightly wider than shoulder-width apart.
Step 2: Lower your body as you would in a regular push-up.
Step 3: As you push yourself up, explode off the ground with enough force to clap your hands together before landing.
Step 4: Quickly place your hands back on the ground to catch yourself and immediately lower back into the next push-up.
Step 5: Continue for the desired number of reps.

Clapping push-ups are excellent for developing explosive strength in your chest, shoulders, and triceps. They also engage your core as you stabilize your body during the explosive movement.

JUMP SQUATS

Jump squats are a powerful lower-body exercise that combines strength with explosive power, targeting your quads, hamstrings, glutes, and calves.

Step 1: Stand with your feet shoulder-width apart, toes pointing slightly outward.
Step 2: Lower yourself into a squat, keeping your chest up and back straight.
Step 3: From the squat position, explode upwards, jumping as high as you can.
Step 4: Land softly on the balls of your feet, immediately lowering back into the squat position.
Step 5: Repeat for the desired number of reps.

Jump squats not only build strength but also improve your explosive power and cardiovascular fitness.

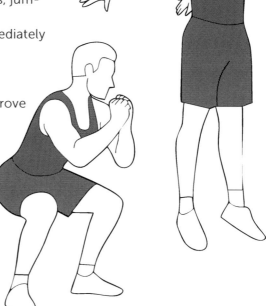

THE NEW CALISTHENICS FORMULA

TUCK JUMPS

Tuck jumps are a high-intensity exercise that targets your entire lower body while engaging your core for stability.

Step 1: Stand with your feet hip-width apart.

Step 2: Bend your knees slightly and jump as high as possible, bringing your knees towards your chest.

Step 3: Keep your arms extended by your sides to help with balance.

Step 4: Land softly on the balls of your feet, quickly absorbing the impact with a slight bend in your knees.

Step 5: Repeat for the desired number of reps.

Tuck jumps are excellent for building explosive power in your legs and improving coordination.

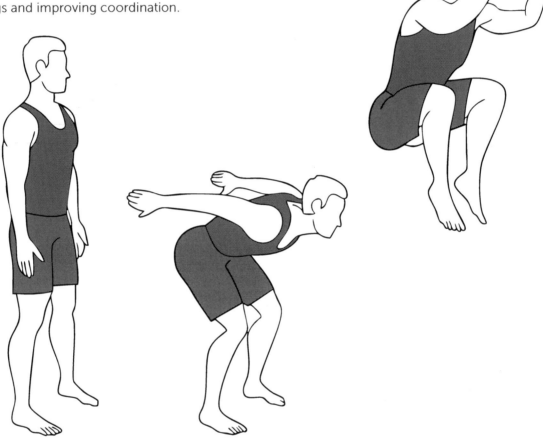

BURPEE BOX JUMPS

This exercise combines the traditional burpee with a box jump, adding an extra challenge to your full-body workout.

Step 1: Stand in front of a sturdy box or bench.

Step 2: Drop into a squat position, place your hands on the ground, and kick your feet back into a plank.

Step 3: Perform a push-up, then jump your feet back towards your hands.

Step 4: Explosively jump onto the box, landing with both feet.

Step 5: Step down from the box and repeat for the desired number of reps.

Burpee box jumps are a great way to combine strength, cardio, and explosive power in one exercise.

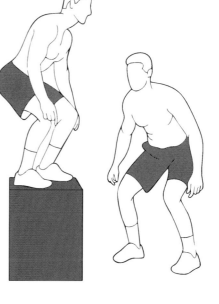

LATERAL BOUNDS

Lateral bounds focus on building explosive power in your legs while improving your agility and coordination.

Step 1: Stand with your feet hip-width apart, knees slightly bent.

Step 2: Push off your right leg, jumping laterally (to the side) as far as you can.

Step 3: Land softly on your left leg, immediately pushing off to jump back to the right.

Step 4: Continue alternating sides, maintaining a quick and controlled movement.

Step 5: Repeat for the desired number of reps.

Lateral bounds engage your glutes, quads, and calves while enhancing lateral (side-to-side) movement.

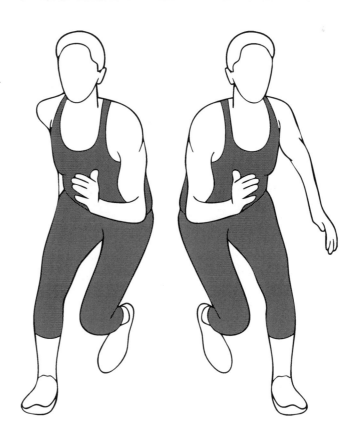

TEMPO CHANGES: SLOWING DOWN FOR STRENGTH

While plyometrics focus on speed and explosiveness, tempo changes emphasize control and muscle endurance by slowing down your movements. This technique increases the time your muscles are under tension, forcing them to work harder throughout the entire range of motion. Slowing down your exercises might sound simple, but it can significantly increase the difficulty and effectiveness of your workout.

SLOW PUSH-UPS

Slow push-ups are a powerful way to build strength in your upper body while improving control and stability.

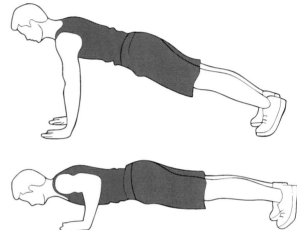

Step 1: Begin in a standard push-up position, keeping your body in a straight line from head to heels.
Step 2: Slowly lower yourself to the ground, taking about three to five seconds to reach the bottom.
Step 3: Pause briefly at the bottom to eliminate any momentum.
Step 4: Push yourself back up just as slowly, focusing on engaging your chest, shoulders, and triceps.
Step 5: Repeat for the desired number of reps.

By slowing down the tempo, you'll engage more muscle fibers, particularly those responsible for stability and control. This makes slow push-ups more challenging than their regular counterparts.

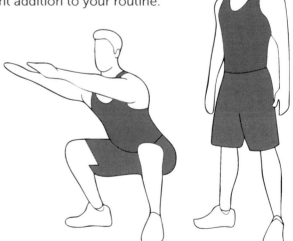

SLOW SQUATS

Slow squats apply the same principle to one of the most fundamental lower-body exercises, making them an excellent addition to your routine.

Step 1: Stand with your feet shoulder-width apart, toes slightly turned out.
Step 2: Slowly lower yourself into a squat, taking about three to five seconds to reach the bottom.
Step 3: Hold the bottom position briefly to eliminate any bounce or momentum.
Step 4: Rise back up just as slowly, focusing on squeezing your glutes and keeping your chest up.
Step 5: Repeat for the desired number of reps.

Slow squats not only target your quads, hamstrings, and glutes but also engage your core as you maintain balance and stability throughout the movement. The slow tempo increases the intensity, making your muscles work harder to control the movement.

SLOW MOUNTAIN CLIMBERS

Slow mountain climbers focus on building core strength, stability, and endurance by slowing down the traditionally fast-paced movement.

Step 1: Start in a plank position with your hands directly under your shoulders and your body in a straight line.
Step 2: Slowly bring your right knee towards your chest, taking about three seconds to complete the movement.
Step 3: Pause for a moment, ensuring your core is engaged.
Step 4: Slowly return your right leg to the starting position, taking another three seconds.
Step 5: Repeat with your left leg, alternating sides for the desired number of reps.

Slowing down mountain climbers increases the time your core muscles are under tension, making this exercise more challenging and effective.

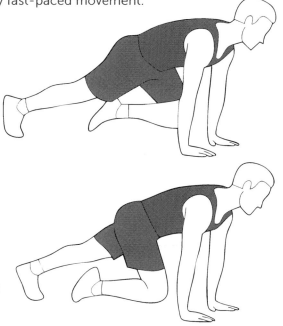

SLOW TRICEPS DIPS

Slow triceps dips emphasize control and strength in your triceps, shoulders, and chest by reducing the speed of each movement.

Step 1: Sit on the edge of a sturdy chair or bench, with your hands gripping the edge and your legs extended out in front of you.
Step 2: Slowly lower your body towards the ground, taking three to five seconds to bend your elbows to a 90-degree angle.
Step 3: Hold the bottom position briefly, keeping tension in your triceps.
Step 4: Slowly push yourself back up to the starting position, taking another three to five seconds.
Step 5: Repeat for the desired number of reps.

This tempo change makes triceps dips more intense, promoting greater muscle engagement and strength development.

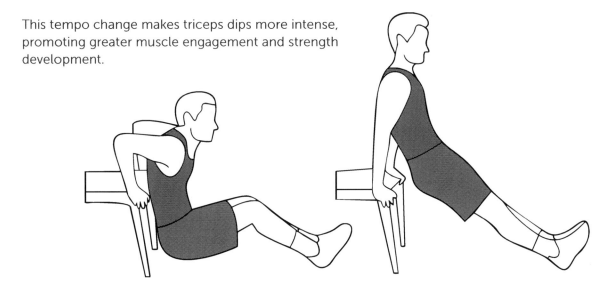

SLOW LEG RAISES

Slow leg raises focus on strengthening your lower abs and hip flexors by controlling the movement speed and maintaining tension.

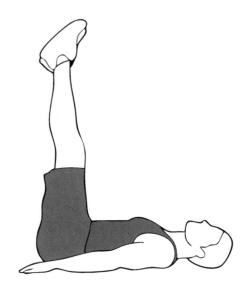

Step 1: Lie flat on your back with your legs extended and your hands at your sides or under your lower back for support.

Step 2: Slowly raise your legs towards the ceiling, taking about three to five seconds to complete the movement.

Step 3: Pause briefly when your legs are perpendicular to the ground.

Step 4: Slowly lower your legs back to the starting position, taking another three to five seconds.

Step 5: Repeat for the desired number of reps.

The slow tempo in leg raises intensifies the exercise, increasing the challenge to your core and helping build abdominal strength.

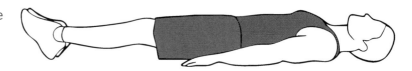

SLOW PLANK WALKOUTS

Slow plank walkouts add an extra challenge to the traditional plank by incorporating slow, controlled movements that engage your entire core.

Step 1: Start in a standing position with your feet hip-width apart.

Step 2: Slowly bend forward at the hips and walk your hands out into a plank position, taking about three to five seconds.

Step 3: Hold the plank position for a few seconds, ensuring your body forms a straight line from head to heels.

Step 4: Slowly walk your hands back towards your feet and return to the standing position, taking another three to five seconds.

Step 5: Repeat for the desired number of reps.

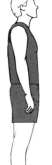

Slowing down plank walkouts increases the time under tension, challenging your core, shoulders, and arms while improving stability and control.

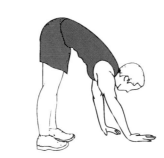
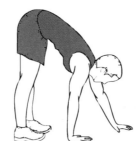
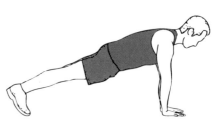

SLOW BICYCLE CRUNCHES

Slow bicycle crunches target your obliques and the entire core by slowing down the movement, ensuring a greater focus on muscle engagement.

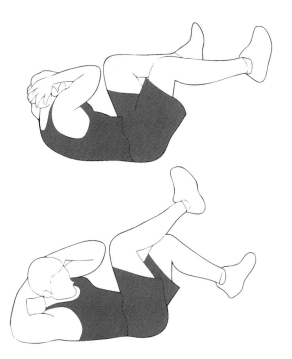

Step 1: Lie on your back with your hands behind your head and your legs raised, knees bent at a 90-degree angle.

Step 2: Slowly bring your right elbow towards your left knee while extending your right leg, taking about three seconds.

Step 3: Pause at the peak of the movement, feeling the contraction in your obliques.

Step 4: Slowly switch sides, bringing your left elbow towards your right knee, taking another three seconds.

Step 5: Continue alternating sides in a controlled manner for the desired number of reps.

By slowing down bicycle crunches, you enhance the intensity and effectiveness of the exercise, building stronger, more defined obliques and abs.

ALTERNATING BETWEEN PLYOMETRICS AND TEMPO CHANGES

To maximize the benefits of your calisthenics routine, consider alternating between plyometric exercises and tempo changes. This combination keeps your workouts dynamic, ensuring that you continue to progress without hitting a plateau. For example, you might start your session with explosive box jumps to fire up your muscles and end with slow squats to build strength and control. By mixing these techniques, you challenge your body in different ways, promoting well-rounded muscle development and preventing boredom.

Incorporating plyometrics and tempo changes into your calisthenics routine is a surefire way to increase the intensity and drive your progress forward. Whether you're aiming to build power, improve endurance, or enhance strength, these methods offer a versatile and effective approach to taking your workout to the next level.

PROGRESSIVE OVERLOAD WITH BODYWEIGHT TRAINING

WHEN YOU START YOUR JOURNEY IN CALISTHENICS, YOU'LL QUICKLY REALIZE THAT BUILDING STRENGTH AND MUSCLE ISN'T JUST ABOUT DOING THE SAME EXERCISES OVER AND OVER. TO TRULY SEE PROGRESS, YOU NEED TO CHALLENGE YOUR MUSCLES IN NEW WAYS. THIS IS WHERE THE CONCEPT OF PROGRESSIVE OVERLOAD COMES INTO PLAY. PROGRESSIVE OVERLOAD MEANS GRADUALLY INCREASING THE DEMANDS ON YOUR BODY, PUSHING IT TO ADAPT AND GROW STRONGER OVER TIME. ALTHOUGH THIS IDEA IS OFTEN LINKED TO WEIGHTLIFTING, IT'S JUST AS CRUCIAL WHEN IT COMES TO BODYWEIGHT EXERCISES.

UNDERSTANDING PROGRESSIVE OVERLOAD IN CALISTHENICS

In the context of calisthenics, progressive overload is about finding ways to make your exercises more challenging as you get stronger. Since you're working with your own body weight, you might think your options are limited. However, there are several effective methods to apply this principle, ensuring that you continue to make gains and avoid plateaus.

INCREASE REPS OR SETS

One of the simplest ways to apply progressive overload is by increasing the number of repetitions or sets you perform. For example, if you're comfortable doing 10 push-ups, aim to do 12 or 15 in your next workout. The same goes for sets—if three sets of 10 push-ups have become easy, try adding a fourth set. By gradually increasing your workload, you force your muscles to adapt to the higher demand, leading to greater strength and endurance.

ADD WEIGHT

As you get stronger, bodyweight exercises that once felt challenging might start to feel too easy. To continue progressing, consider adding extra weight. This doesn't mean you need to head to the gym and start lifting dumbbells. Instead, you can use a weighted vest or simply wear a backpack filled with some books or other heavy items. Adding weight increases the resistance your muscles have to work against, making the exercises more challenging and effective.

For example, if you're doing bodyweight squats and find that they're no longer pushing you, put on a weighted vest or backpack and try the squats again. You'll notice that the extra weight makes a significant difference, forcing your muscles to work harder and promoting further strength gains.

USE ADVANCED VARIATIONS

Another way to incorporate progressive overload is by transitioning to more advanced variations of the exercises you're already doing. As you become proficient in basic movements, challenging yourself with more difficult variations can keep your progress moving forward.

Take push-ups, for example. If regular push-ups have become too easy, you can move to diamond push-ups, where your hands are placed close together under your chest, increasing the intensity on your triceps and chest. Similarly, if bodyweight squats no longer feel challenging, you can progress to pistol squats, a single-leg squat that requires significant strength, balance, and coordination.

THE IMPORTANCE OF CONSISTENCY

The key to successfully implementing progressive overload is consistency. It's not about making huge leaps from one workout to the next but rather about making small, sustainable improvements over time. For instance, instead of trying to jump from 10 push-ups to 50 in one session, focus on adding just a couple of reps each week. These incremental changes might seem small at first, but they add up over time, leading to significant progress in your strength and muscle development.

Consistency also means paying attention to your body and giving it the time it needs to adapt. Progressive overload isn't just about pushing harder—it's also about allowing your muscles to recover and grow stronger. By gradually increasing the challenge and sticking with your routine, you'll find that your body adapts, your strength increases, and you're able to tackle more advanced calisthenics exercises with confidence.

SAMPLE INTERMEDIATE WORKOUT PLAN: FULL-BODY AND SPLIT ROUTINES

AS YOU ADVANCE IN YOUR CALISTHENICS JOURNEY, IT'S ESSENTIAL TO HAVE A WELL-STRUCTURED WORKOUT PLAN THAT CHALLENGES YOUR BODY WHILE PROMOTING STEADY PROGRESS. TRANSITIONING FROM BEGINNER TO INTERMEDIATE EXERCISES REQUIRES MORE STRATEGIC PLANNING TO ENSURE THAT YOU'RE TARGETING ALL MAJOR MUSCLE GROUPS EFFECTIVELY. THIS SECTION INTRODUCES A SAMPLE INTERMEDIATE WORKOUT PLAN, OFFERING BOTH FULL-BODY AND SPLIT ROUTINES THAT YOU CAN INCORPORATE INTO YOUR WEEKLY SCHEDULE. THESE ROUTINES ARE DESIGNED TO PUSH YOUR LIMITS, IMPROVE YOUR STRENGTH, AND HELP YOU ACHIEVE YOUR FITNESS GOALS.

FULL-BODY ROUTINE

A full-body routine is an excellent option if you prefer to work all major muscle groups in one session. This routine should be performed three times a week, with at least one day of rest between each session to allow your muscles to recover and grow stronger.

- **Warm-Up (5-10 minutes):** Begin with dynamic stretching or light cardio exercises such as jumping jacks, high knees, or butt kicks. This helps to increase your heart rate, loosen up your muscles, and prepare your body for the workout ahead.

- **Push-Ups (Diamond or Archer):** Perform 3 sets of 10-12 reps. Diamond push-ups target your triceps and inner chest, while archer push-ups add an element of unilateral training, working each side of your body independently. Both variations are great for building upper body strength and endurance.

- **Pull-Ups or Chin-Ups:** Do 3 sets of 8-10 reps. Pull-ups primarily target your back muscles, particularly the lats, while chin-ups emphasize your biceps. These exercises are crucial for developing upper body pulling strength.

- **Parallel Bar Dips:** Complete 3 sets of 10-12 reps. Dips are highly effective for working your triceps, chest, and shoulders. Using parallel bars allows for a greater range of motion, making the exercise more challenging.

- **Pistol Squats:** Perform 3 sets of 6-8 reps per leg. Pistol squats are a challenging single-leg exercise that targets your quads, hamstrings, glutes, and core. They require balance, strength, and flexibility, making them a staple in any advanced calisthenics routine.

- **Hanging Leg Raises:** Do 3 sets of 10-12 reps. This exercise is excellent for developing core strength, particularly in the lower abs. Hanging leg raises also engage your hip flexors and grip strength.

- **Box Jumps:** Finish with 3 sets of 10-12 reps. Box jumps are a powerful plyometric exercise that builds explosive strength in your legs and improves your cardiovascular endurance. Ensure you land softly to reduce the impact on your joints.

- **Cool Down (5-10 minutes):** End your workout with static stretching, focusing on the muscles you've worked. This helps to improve flexibility, reduce muscle tension, and promote recovery.

UPPER/LOWER SPLIT ROUTINE

If you prefer to split your workouts, the following two-day routine is designed to target your upper and lower body on different days. Perform each workout twice a week, with a rest day in between.

DAY 1 UPPER BODY

- **Warm-Up (5-10 minutes):** Start with dynamic stretching or light cardio to prepare your upper body for the workout.

- **Diamond Push-Ups:** Do 4 sets of 10-12 reps. This variation of push-ups focuses on your triceps and inner chest, providing a greater challenge than regular push-ups.

- **Pull-Ups or Chin-Ups:** Perform 4 sets of 8-10 reps. These exercises are essential for building upper body strength, targeting your back and biceps.

- **Parallel Bar Dips:** Complete 4 sets of 10-12 reps. Dips are effective for strengthening your triceps, chest, and shoulders.

- **Hanging Leg Raises:** Do 4 sets of 10-12 reps. This exercise targets your core, helping to build strong and defined abs.

- **Clapping Push-Ups:** Finish with 3 sets of 8-10 reps. Clapping push-ups are a plyometric variation that increases the intensity, focusing on explosive power in your chest, shoulders, and triceps.

- **Cool Down (5-10 minutes):** Conclude with static stretching to relax your muscles and aid in recovery.

DAY 2 LOWER BODY

- **Warm-Up (5-10 minutes):** Begin with dynamic stretching or light cardio to warm up your lower body.

- **Pistol Squats:** Perform 4 sets of 6-8 reps per leg. These single-leg squats are highly effective for building leg strength and improving balance.

- **Jump Squats:** Do 4 sets of 10-12 reps. Jump squats are a plyometric exercise that adds an explosive element to your lower body workout, targeting your quads, hamstrings, and glutes.

- **Slow Squats:** Complete 3 sets of 8-10 reps. Slow squats increase the time under tension, making the exercise more challenging and effective for building strength.

- **Box Jumps:** Finish with 3 sets of 10-12 reps. This exercise develops explosive leg power and improves overall athleticism.

- **Cool Down (5-10 minutes):** End your session with static stretching, focusing on the muscles worked during the routine.

ADJUSTING YOUR WORKOUTS

As you get stronger, don't hesitate to adjust your workouts. If a particular exercise becomes too easy, increase the difficulty by adding reps, sets, or weight or by progressing to a more advanced variation. On the other hand, if you're struggling with a certain move, there's no shame in scaling back or modifying the exercise until you're ready to progress. The key is to find the balance between challenging yourself and respecting your body's limits.

RECOVERY AND REST

Rest is just as important as the workouts themselves. Your muscles need time to recover and rebuild after each session, so make sure you're getting enough rest between workouts. Incorporating active recovery days—where you do light activities like walking, stretching, or yoga—can help improve your recovery while keeping you moving.

THE BOTTOM LINE

Moving into intermediate calisthenics is an exciting step in your fitness journey. It's where you'll begin to see real transformation—not just in your strength and endurance, but in your confidence and sense of accomplishment. Remember, calisthenics isn't just about the physical benefits; it's about mastering your body and unlocking your potential.

So, embrace the journey. Stay consistent, be patient with yourself, and celebrate every milestone, no matter how small. You've already come so far, and the best is yet to come.

ADVANCED CALISTHENICS MASTERY

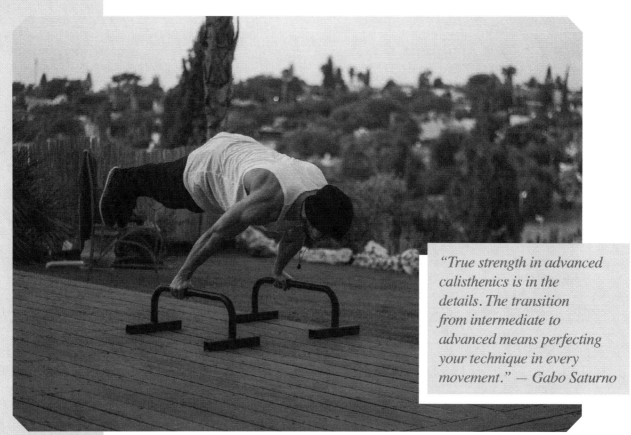

> *"True strength in advanced calisthenics is in the details. The transition from intermediate to advanced means perfecting your technique in every movement."* — Gabo Saturno

Imagine being able to lift your body with ease, defying gravity in ways that seem impossible to most. That's the power of advanced calisthenics. If you've mastered the basics, it's time to step up. This chapter is all about pushing past your limits, both mentally and physically, to conquer movements that require true mastery.

You'll dive into advanced upper and lower body exercises like muscle-ups, pistol squats, and one-arm push-ups. We'll also take your core strength to a whole new level, teaching you how to build the control needed for static holds like the human flag or planche. But don't worry—it's all broken down step by step. Progressions will help you build the strength and skill required to tackle each movement safely.

By the end of this chapter, you'll also learn how to create advanced routines that balance strength, skill, and mobility. It's about building a solid foundation while continuously challenging yourself. Remember, the key is patience, consistency, and perfecting your form. Ready to level up?

MOVING BEYOND BASICS: THE JOURNEY TO ADVANCED MOVEMENTS

YOU'VE PUT IN THE WORK. THE BASICS ARE NO LONGER A CHALLENGE. PUSH-UPS, PULL-UPS, SQUATS, AND PLANKS ARE PART OF YOUR DAILY ROUTINE. NOW, YOU'RE READY TO TAKE YOUR CALISTHENICS JOURNEY TO THE NEXT LEVEL. BUT MOVING FROM BASIC TO ADVANCED CALISTHENICS ISN'T JUST ABOUT ADDING MORE REPS OR MAKING EXERCISES HARDER. IT'S ABOUT A COMPLETE TRANSFORMATION IN HOW YOU APPROACH YOUR TRAINING, BOTH MENTALLY AND PHYSICALLY. YOU'RE ABOUT TO STEP INTO A WORLD WHERE STRENGTH MEETS SKILL, WHERE EVERY MOVEMENT IS A TEST OF YOUR MASTERY OVER YOUR OWN BODY. AND IN THIS CHAPTER, YOU'LL LEARN EXACTLY HOW TO MAKE THAT LEAP.

To excel in advanced calisthenics, you need more than just physical strength; mental toughness is equally crucial. The exercises you're about to encounter are complex and demanding. They require a blend of raw power, precise coordination, and, most importantly, patience. It's not uncommon to hit a plateau or face frustration when progress seems slow. But this is where the true mastery begins—pushing through those barriers, staying disciplined, and keeping your eyes on the long-term goal. Every advanced movement you learn will not only enhance your physical abilities but also sharpen your mental focus and resilience.

Advanced calisthenics is a journey that challenges your entire being. It's not just about doing more—it's about doing better, with a deeper understanding of your body's capabilities and limitations. Each movement becomes an art form where execution is as important as power. You'll be exploring exercises that demand impeccable technique, and the journey to mastering them will transform you, both in body and in mind. So, let's dive into the world of advanced calisthenics and discover the true potential of your body.

ADVANCED UPPER BODY EXERCISES

EVER TRIED A PUSH-UP THAT FEELS LIKE YOU'RE DEFYING GRAVITY? ADVANCED UPPER BODY EXERCISES PUSH YOUR STRENGTH AND BALANCE TO THE NEXT LEVEL. IN THIS SECTION, YOU'LL MASTER MOVES LIKE MUSCLE-UPS, ONE-ARM PUSH-UPS, AND HANDSTAND PUSH-UPS. YOU'LL ALSO LEARN HOW TO BUILD UP TO IMPRESSIVE SKILLS LIKE THE PLANCHE, ALL WHILE WORKING ON CONTROL AND COORDINATION. THESE EXERCISES AREN'T JUST ABOUT BRUTE STRENGTH—THEY CHALLENGE YOUR ENTIRE BODY. READY TO TEST YOUR LIMITS AND TAKE YOUR UPPER BODY WORKOUTS TO NEW HEIGHTS? LET'S GET STARTED!

MUSCLE-UPS

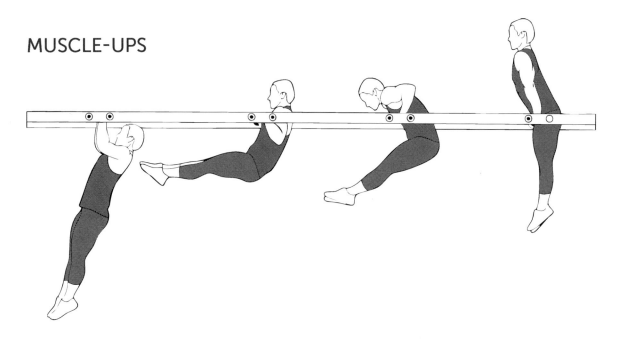

When you think of advanced calisthenics, the muscle-up stands out as a true test of your strength, agility, and technique. This move isn't just about pulling yourself up and over the bar; it's about executing a powerful, fluid motion that combines elements of both the pull-up and the dip. Mastering the muscle-up will put you in an elite group of athletes who have conquered one of the most challenging and rewarding exercises in calisthenics.

HOW TO PERFORM A MUSCLE-UP

Here's how you can break down the muscle-up into manageable steps:

1. **Start with a strong pull-up:** Grip the bar slightly wider than shoulder-width. Hang from the bar with your arms fully extended and your body straight. Engage your core and pull yourself up explosively, aiming to bring your chest as high as possible—ideally above the bar.

2. **Transition phase:** As you reach the peak of your pull-up, begin to rotate your wrists forward so your palms face downward. Simultaneously, lean your chest over the bar, transitioning from a pulling to a pushing motion. This is the trickiest part, requiring both timing and coordination.

3. **Push to finish:** Once your chest is over the bar, press down firmly as if performing a dip. Extend your arms fully to push your body above the bar. At this point, your body should be in a straight line above the bar, completing the muscle-up.

With consistent practice and attention to detail, you'll be able to conquer the muscle-up. Remember, it's not just about brute force but also about smooth execution and control. As you refine your technique, you'll find the muscle-up becoming more natural, allowing you to perform this iconic movement with confidence and ease.

ONE-ARM PUSH-UPS AND PULL-UPS

When it comes to demonstrating raw upper body strength, few exercises rival the one-arm push-up and one-arm pull-up. These movements are more than just feats of power; they require exceptional balance, stability, and control. Mastering these advanced calisthenics exercises not only showcases your physical prowess but also significantly enhances your functional strength, making you more capable in a variety of athletic pursuits.

HOW TO PERFORM A ONE-ARM PUSH-UP

Achieving a one-arm push-up requires both strength and technique. Here's how to approach it:

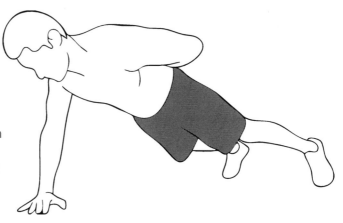

1. **Build a solid foundation:** Ensure you can perform at least 20 perfect form regular push-ups. This ensures your chest, shoulders, triceps, and core are strong enough to handle the transition to one-arm push-ups.

2. **Archer push-ups:** Begin training with archer push-ups where one arm assists the other by extending out to the side. Gradually shift more weight to the working arm by reducing the amount of assistance provided by the other arm.

3. **Elevated one-arm push-ups:** Place your working hand on an elevated surface (e.g., a bench or step). Keep your body straight and core tight, and lower your chest towards the surface while maintaining balance. As you get stronger, progressively lower the height of the elevated surface until you can perform the push-up on the ground.

4. **Full one-arm push-up:** With feet spread slightly wider than shoulder-width, place one hand behind your back or by your side. Lower your body in a controlled manner, ensuring your hips don't sag or twist. Push back up, keeping your body as a single, stable unit.

HOW TO PERFORM A ONE-ARM PULL-UP

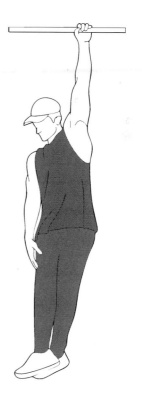

One-arm pull-ups are a significant challenge, even for experienced athletes. Follow these steps to build up to this impressive movement:

1. **Start with assisted one-arm pull-ups:** Use a resistance band to assist you by looping it over the bar and placing one foot inside the band. Alternatively, grip the bar with both hands but focus on pulling more with the working arm.

2. **Archer pull-ups:** Once your pulling strength improves, transition to archer pull-ups. Similar to archer push-ups, one arm performs the pull while the other assists by holding onto the bar or another object at an angle. This helps develop the unilateral strength needed for the full one-arm pull-up.

3. **Negative one-arm pull-ups:** Jump or use a step to get your chin above the bar with one arm. Slowly lower yourself down, focusing on controlling the descent. This eccentric phase builds the strength necessary for the upward motion.

4. **Full one-arm pull-up:** Grip the bar with one hand, keeping your other arm close to your body. Engage your core and pull yourself up, aiming to bring your chin above the bar. Maintain control throughout the movement, avoiding any swinging or excessive use of momentum.

Achieving the one-arm push-up and pull-up marks a significant milestone in your calisthenics journey. These movements are not only impressive but also provide a solid foundation for further advanced exercises. Stay committed, keep practicing, and enjoy the process of becoming stronger and more skilled in your calisthenics mastery.

PLANCHE PROGRESSIONS

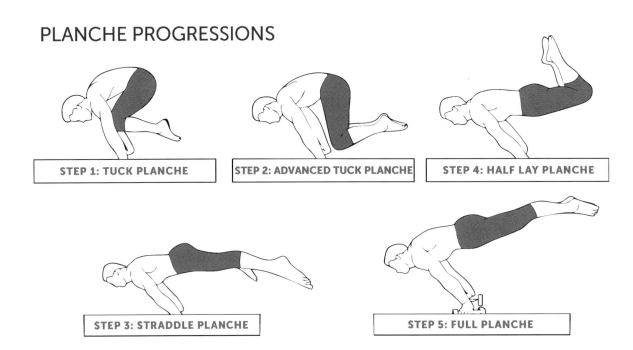

| STEP 1: TUCK PLANCHE | STEP 2: ADVANCED TUCK PLANCHE | STEP 4: HALF LAY PLANCHE |

| STEP 3: STRADDLE PLANCHE | STEP 5: FULL PLANCHE |

The planche is a true showcase of strength, control, and balance in calisthenics. Achieving a full planche is a milestone that requires not just upper body power but also a rock-solid core and impeccable technique. While the planche might seem daunting at first, breaking it down into smaller, manageable progressions makes this advanced skill attainable. Let's explore the journey to mastering the planche, step by step.

HOW TO PROGRESS TOWARD A FULL PLANCHE

Progressing to a full planche involves mastering a series of exercises that gradually build the required strength and technique. Here's how to approach each stage:

1. **Planche Lean:** Start by positioning yourself in a push-up stance with your hands shoulder-width apart. Lean your body forward, shifting your weight onto your hands while keeping your arms straight. The goal is to increase the lean angle over time, feeling the load transfer more to your shoulders and chest. Focus on keeping a hollow body position, where your lower back is slightly rounded, and your core is engaged.

2. **Tuck Planche:** Once you're comfortable with the planche lean, move on to the tuck planche. From the planche lean position, tuck your knees into your chest while balancing on your hands. Keep your arms straight and engage your core to maintain stability. The tuck planche is challenging because it shifts more of your body weight onto your arms, requiring greater upper body strength.

3. **Advanced Tuck Planche:** In this progression, slightly extend your legs from the tuck position, making it more challenging. The advanced tuck planche increases the lever arm, placing more stress on your shoulders and core. Continue to focus on keeping your arms straight and maintaining the hollow body position.

4. **Straddle Planche:** After mastering the advanced tuck, move on to the straddle planche. From the tuck position, gradually extend your legs outward into a straddle, spreading them apart to reduce the lever effect. This progression demands even more strength and balance as your legs are extended, increasing the load on your shoulders. Aim to keep your legs as straight as possible and continue to engage your core to hold the position.

5. **Full Planche:** The final progression is the full planche, where you hold your body parallel to the ground with your legs fully extended. To achieve this, bring your legs together from the straddle position, maintaining straight arms and a hollow body. This requires maximal strength, stability, and control across your entire body. It's important to keep practicing the earlier progressions even as you attempt the full planche to maintain strength and prevent injury.

Achieving the planche is a testament to your dedication and hard work in calisthenics. It's a skill that requires a blend of strength, technique, and mental focus, making it one of the most rewarding accomplishments in bodyweight training. As you continue to progress, you'll not only build impressive physical strength but also a deeper connection with your body and its capabilities.

HANDSTAND PUSH-UPS

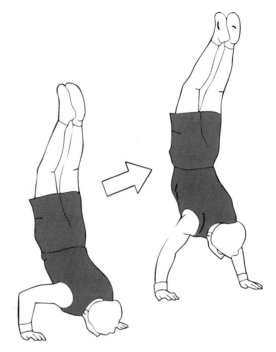

Handstand push-ups represent a pinnacle in bodyweight training, combining the traditional push-up's power with the added challenge of balancing your entire body upside down. This advanced move demands not only significant upper body strength but also excellent coordination and balance. Mastering handstand push-ups is a rewarding goal that showcases your calisthenics progress and pushes your physical limits.

HOW TO PROGRESS TOWARD HANDSTAND PUSH-UPS

Progressing to a full handstand push-up involves several stages, each designed to build the necessary strength, balance, and technique. Here's how to approach it:

1. **Freestanding Handstand:** Before attempting handstand push-ups, ensure you can hold a freestanding handstand for at least 30 seconds. Practice by kicking up into a handstand against a wall, then gradually move away from the wall as your balance improves. Focus on maintaining a tight core, straight arms, and a neutral head position to keep your body aligned.

2. **Pike Push-Ups:** Begin with pike push-ups to develop the shoulder strength needed for handstand push-ups. Start in a downward dog position with your hips raised and your hands and feet on the ground. Lower your head toward the ground by bending your elbows, then push back up to the starting position. The pike push-up mimics the movement pattern of a handstand push-up but with your feet on the ground, making it an excellent progression exercise.

3. **Wall-Assisted Handstand Push-Ups:** Once you're comfortable with pike push-ups, transition to wall-assisted handstand push-ups. Kick up into a handstand with your back facing the wall and your hands placed shoulder-width apart on the ground. Lower your head slowly toward the ground by bending your elbows, then press back up to the starting position. Keep your core tight and avoid arching your back to maintain stability and control.

4. **Negative Handstand Push-Ups:** As you build strength, start practicing negatives to develop the control needed for freestanding handstand push-ups. Kick up into a freestanding handstand and slowly lower yourself to the ground, focusing on maintaining balance and control throughout the movement. This eccentric phase helps build the strength required to press back up into a handstand.

5. **Freestanding Handstand Push-Ups:** The ultimate goal is to perform freestanding handstand push-ups without any wall support. Start in a freestanding handstand position and slowly lower your head toward the ground, keeping your body aligned and controlled. Push back up to the starting position, using your shoulders and triceps to complete the movement. This exercise is extremely challenging and requires not only strength but also precise balance and coordination.

THE NEW CALISTHENICS FORMULA

Achieving freestanding handstand push-ups is a significant milestone in calisthenics, demonstrating your dedication and hard work. This move not only strengthens your upper body but also enhances your balance and body control, making it a valuable addition to your calisthenics skill set. With patience, persistence, and a focus on technique, you'll soon be able to perform handstand push-ups with confidence and ease.

ADVANCED LOWER BODY EXERCISES

EVER TRIED BALANCING ON ONE LEG WHILE LOWERING YOURSELF TO THE GROUND? ADVANCED LOWER BODY EXERCISES LIKE SHRIMP SQUATS AND JUMPING LUNGES PUSH YOUR LEGS AND CORE BEYOND THE USUAL. IN THIS SECTION, YOU'LL DIVE INTO SHRIMP SQUATS, SINGLE-LEG LEVERS, AND PLYOMETRICS TO BUILD EXPLOSIVE STRENGTH AND STABILITY. THESE EXERCISES ARE DESIGNED TO BOOST YOUR BALANCE, POWER, AND ENDURANCE. IF YOU'RE READY TO PUSH YOUR LOWER BODY TO ITS PEAK PERFORMANCE, THIS IS WHERE THE REAL WORK BEGINS!

SHRIMP SQUATS AND SINGLE-LEG LEVERS

When it comes to advanced lower body exercises, shrimp squats and single-leg levers (also known as pistol squats) are at the top of the list. These movements are not just about brute strength; they also demand balance, flexibility, and mobility. Mastering these exercises can significantly enhance your lower body power, stability, and overall athleticism, making them essential additions to any serious calisthenics or strength training regimen.

HOW TO PERFORM A SHRIMP SQUAT

The shrimp squat, also known as the airborne lunge, is a powerful exercise for building leg strength and improving balance. Here's how to approach it:

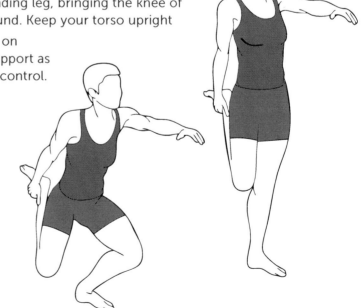

1. **Start with assisted shrimp squats:** Stand on one leg with the other leg bent behind you, holding onto a stable surface for support. Slowly lower your body by bending your standing leg, bringing the knee of the non-working leg close to the ground. Keep your torso upright and your working leg stable, focusing on controlling the movement. Use the support as needed to help maintain balance and control.

2. **Progress to unassisted shrimp squats:** Once you're comfortable with the assisted variation, try performing the movement without holding onto anything. Focus on maintaining balance throughout the movement by engaging your core and keeping your eyes fixed on a point in front of you. Lower yourself slowly and with control, ensuring that your knee nearly touches the ground.

3. Increase the difficulty: To add more challenge, hold a weight in front of you while performing the shrimp squat. Alternatively, slow down the lowering phase to increase the time under tension, which will further strengthen your muscles and improve your balance.

HOW TO PERFORM A SINGLE-LEG LEVER (PISTOL SQUAT)

The pistol squat is another advanced lower-body movement that requires strength, flexibility, and balance. Here's how to progress toward mastering it:

1. **Start with assisted pistol squats:** Stand on one leg with the other leg extended straight in front of you. Hold onto a support (like a pole or a doorframe) to help maintain balance as you lower yourself into a squat. Focus on keeping your chest up, your core engaged, and your extended leg as straight as possible. Lower yourself slowly, aiming to bring your hips below your knee before pushing back up to the starting position.

2. **Work on ankle mobility and hamstring flexibility:** Ankle mobility and hamstring flexibility are often limiting factors in performing a full pistol squat. Incorporate stretches and mobility drills into your routine to improve these areas, making the pistol squat more accessible. Calf stretches, deep squats, and hamstring stretches are particularly useful.

3. **Progress to freestanding pistol squats:** As you gain strength and flexibility, start practicing pistol squats without any assistance. Lower yourself in a controlled manner, focusing on keeping your torso upright and your extended leg straight. Aim for a smooth, controlled movement throughout the entire range of motion.

4. **Increase the challenge:** Once you've mastered the basic pistol squat, you can add weight or slow down the movement to make it more challenging. Holding a kettlebell or dumbbell in front of you can help counterbalance your body, making the movement slightly easier while increasing the load on your leg muscles.

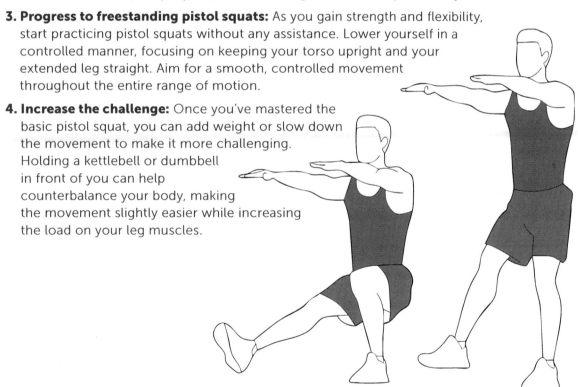

Shrimp squats and single-leg levers are advanced exercises that offer immense benefits for your lower body strength and stability. They challenge your muscles in unique ways, pushing you to develop greater control and balance. As you work through the progressions, you'll not only build impressive leg strength but also enhance your overall athletic performance. With dedication and consistency, these exercises will become a powerful tool in your fitness arsenal.

JUMPING LUNGES AND OTHER PLYOMETRIC EXERCISES

Plyometric exercises are a cornerstone of athletic training, offering a unique blend of strength, speed, and agility. Among these exercises, jumping lunges stand out for their ability to build explosive power in the legs while also enhancing coordination and balance. Incorporating jumping lunges and other plyometric movements into your routine can significantly elevate your lower body strength and overall athleticism.

<u>HOW TO PERFORM JUMPING LUNGES</u>

Jumping lunges requires a combination of strength, balance, and coordination. Here's how to master them:

1. **Start with regular lunges:** Begin by performing standard lunges to build the necessary strength and stability in your legs. Step forward with one leg, lowering your hips until both knees are bent at a 90-degree angle. Keep your torso upright and your core engaged. Push off your front foot to return to the starting position, then switch legs.

2. **Add a small jump:** Once you're comfortable with regular lunges, incorporate a small jump as you switch legs. From the lunge position, push off explosively with both feet, switching your legs in mid-air. Land softly in a lunge position with the opposite leg forward, absorbing the impact through your legs.

3. **Increase the height and intensity:** As your power and coordination improve, focus on increasing the height of your jump. Aim for a controlled, explosive movement, ensuring you maintain proper form throughout the exercise. Keep your core engaged and your movements smooth to avoid injury.

4. **Focus on soft landings:** One of the key aspects of jumping lunges is landing softly to reduce the impact on your joints. As you land, bend your knees slightly and engage your muscles to absorb the shock. Control your descent into the lunge position, making sure your knees track over your toes.

<u>DEPTH JUMPS</u>

Depth jumps are a high-intensity plyometric exercise that focuses on developing explosive power and strength in your lower body. This exercise also improves your ability to absorb impact and quickly transition into an upward movement, which is essential for sports that require quick bursts of power.

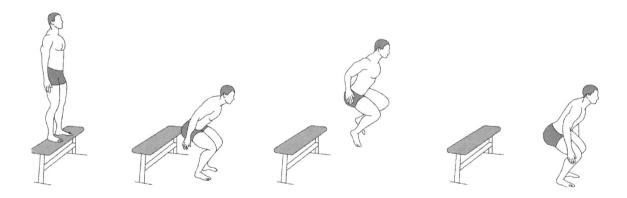

How to Perform:

• Start by standing on a sturdy platform or box that is about 12-24 inches high.

• Step off the platform with one foot, allowing your body to drop to the ground naturally.

• As soon as you land, immediately jump as high as possible, focusing on minimizing ground contact time.

• Use your arms to help generate momentum by swinging them upward as you jump.

• Land softly on the ground, bending your knees to absorb the impact, and then stand up to return to the starting position.

Depth jumps are an effective way to build explosive power in your legs, improve your vertical jump, and enhance your ability to quickly generate force. Incorporate them into your training routine to take your lower body strength and athleticism to the next level.

SINGLE-LEG BOX JUMPS

Single-leg box jumps are a challenging variation of the traditional box jump that requires exceptional balance, coordination, and unilateral leg strength. This exercise targets each leg individually, helping to correct imbalances and enhance explosive power.

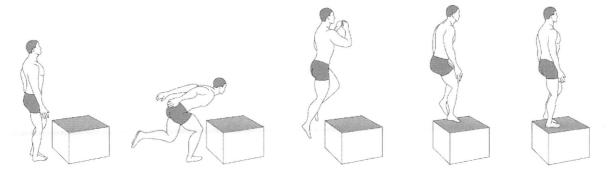

How to Perform:

• Stand in front of a sturdy box or platform that is about 12-18 inches high.

• Balance on one leg, with your other leg slightly bent and lifted off the ground.

• Lower yourself into a slight squat on your standing leg, then explosively push off the ground to jump onto the box, landing softly on the same leg.

• Focus on using your arms for momentum and maintaining balance throughout the movement.

• Step down from the box with both feet and repeat on the other leg.

Single-leg box jumps are an excellent exercise for building unilateral leg strength, improving balance, and enhancing your overall power. They are particularly beneficial for athletes who need to generate force from one leg, such as sprinters or jumpers.

DEPTH DROP TO BROAD JUMP

This combination exercise pairs the depth drop with a broad jump to develop both vertical and horizontal power. It's an advanced plyometric drill that enhances your ability to absorb impact and immediately transition into a powerful jump.

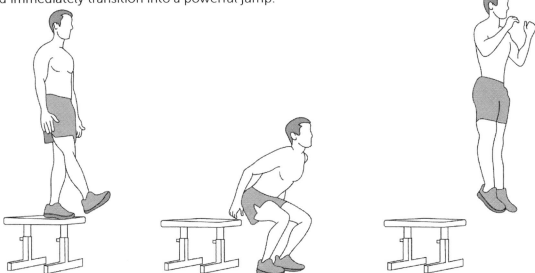

How to Perform:

• Start by standing on a platform or box that is 12-24 inches high.

• Step off the platform, landing softly on both feet.

• As soon as you land, immediately perform a broad jump by pushing off the ground and jumping forward as far as possible.

• Focus on landing softly with both feet and maintaining balance upon landing.

• Stand up and return to the starting position to repeat the exercise.

Depth drop to broad jump is an effective way to build explosive power in both vertical and horizontal planes. This exercise is ideal for athletes who need to develop quick, powerful movements in multiple directions, such as football players or basketball players.

SPLIT SQUAT JUMPS

Split squat jumps are a plyometric exercise that targets the quads, hamstrings, glutes, and calves. This movement is excellent for developing explosive power, leg endurance, and coordination, especially in a unilateral context.

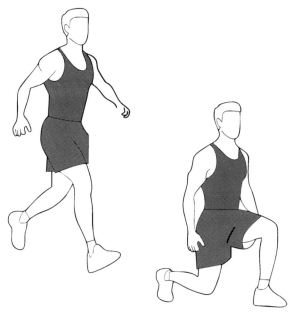

How to Perform:

• Begin in a lunge position with one foot forward and the other foot behind you; both knees should be bent at 90 degrees.

•Push off the ground explosively with both legs, jumping as high as possible.

• While in the air, switch the position of your legs so that you land in a lunge with the opposite leg forward.

• Focus on landing softly and maintaining your balance throughout the movement.

• Immediately jump again, repeating the movement in a continuous, controlled manner.

Split squat jumps are a dynamic exercise that builds explosive power, improves coordination, and increases lower body strength. They're particularly beneficial for athletes who perform activities that require rapid directional changes and unilateral leg strength.

POWER SKIPPING

Power skipping is an advanced plyometric drill that involves exaggerated skipping motions to develop explosive leg strength, coordination, and overall lower body power. This exercise mimics the movements of bounding but incorporates a rhythmic, skipping motion for additional challenge and variety.

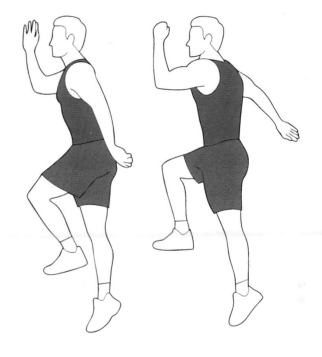

How to Perform:

• Start by standing with your feet shoulder-width apart.

• Push off the ground with one foot, driving your opposite knee high into the air while swinging your arms to generate momentum.

• As you land on the same foot, immediately push off again and repeat the movement with the opposite leg.

• Focus on driving your knees high, maintaining a rhythm, and pushing off the ground as powerfully as possible.

• Continue skipping forward for a set distance or number of repetitions.

Power skipping is a fun and effective way to develop explosive power, coordination, and rhythm in your lower body. It's particularly useful for athletes in sports that require sprinting, jumping, and quick changes of direction, such as soccer, track and field, or basketball.

BOUNDING

Bounding is an advanced plyometric exercise that mimics exaggerated running strides. It focuses on developing explosive power, leg strength, and coordination by pushing off the ground with maximum force and driving the knees high with each stride. Bounding is often used by athletes to improve sprinting speed, jumping ability, and overall lower body power.

How to Perform:

• Start in a standing position with your feet shoulder-width apart and your body slightly leaning forward.

• Begin by pushing off explosively with one foot, driving your opposite knee high into the air as you leap forward.

• Land softly on the opposite foot, immediately pushing off again with the same intensity to continue the movement.

• Focus on extending your stride as far as possible with each bound, maintaining a rhythm, and driving your knees high.

• Keep your core engaged and your arms swinging naturally to help generate momentum.

• Perform the exercise for a set distance or number of repetitions, ensuring each stride is powerful and controlled.

Bounding is an excellent exercise for enhancing leg strength, speed, and coordination. It's particularly beneficial for athletes who need to develop explosive power and improve their performance in sports that require sprinting, jumping, or rapid changes in direction. By incorporating bounding into your training routine, you'll build the necessary strength and agility to excel in a variety of athletic endeavors.

Lower-body plyometric exercises are powerful tools for building explosive leg strength, agility, and coordination. By incorporating these movements into your routine, you'll not only improve your athletic performance but also develop a more balanced and resilient lower body. With consistent practice and attention to form, you'll see significant gains in your power, speed, and overall fitness.

CORE STRENGTH TO THE NEXT LEVEL

READY TO TAKE YOUR CORE STRENGTH BEYOND THE BASICS? ADVANCED MOVES LIKE FRONT LE-
VERS, DRAGON FLAGS, AND L-SITS WILL PUSH YOUR CORE TO NEW HEIGHTS. IN THIS SECTION,
YOU'LL LEARN HOW TO MASTER THESE CHALLENGING EXERCISES THAT REQUIRE FULL-BODY CON-
TROL AND SERIOUS STABILITY. FROM FRONT LEVERS TO V-SITS, THESE MOVES AREN'T JUST ABOUT
A STRONG CORE—THEY TEST YOUR BALANCE AND ENDURANCE, TOO. GET READY TO FEEL THE BURN
AND BUILD CORE STRENGTH LIKE NEVER BEFORE!

FRONT LEVER AND BACK LEVER

The front lever and back lever are two iconic static holds in calisthenics that test your core
strength, stability, and control to the extreme. These advanced movements require not only
immense strength but also precision and body awareness. Successfully executing these exercises is a testament to your progress in calisthenics, as they engage multiple muscle groups,
including your lats, lower back, abs, and shoulders. Let's explore how to progress towards
mastering these challenging skills.

HOW TO PERFORM THE FRONT LEVER

The front lever is a demanding exercise that requires a step-by-step approach to build up the
necessary strength and technique. Here's how to progress towards it:

1. **Tuck Lever Hold:** Begin by hanging from a pull-up bar with your arms straight and your
   body fully extended. Tuck your knees to your chest, engaging your core to lift your hips until
   your back is parallel to the ground. Hold this position, keeping your body in a tight ball and
   maintaining a hollow body posture (slight posterior pelvic tilt). This exercise strengthens
   your core and lats, helping you develop the initial strength needed for the front lever.

2. **Advanced Tuck Lever:** Once you can hold the tuck lever for 20-30 seconds, progress to
   the advanced tuck. From the tuck position, extend your hips slightly so that your thighs are
   parallel to the ground, but keep your knees bent. This variation increases the difficulty by
   extending the lever arm, placing more stress on your core and lats.

3. **Straddle Front Lever:** When you've mastered the advanced tuck, move on to the straddle
   front lever. Extend your legs outward into a straddle position while keeping them straight. The
   straddle reduces the leverage compared to a full front lever, making it a great intermediate
   step. Focus on keeping your body aligned and your core engaged to maintain the position.

4. **Full Front Lever:** The final step is the full front lever, where you hold your body completely
   horizontal with your legs together and fully extended. Engage your core, lats, and lower
   back to maintain the hollow body position, keeping your body as straight as possible. This
   position demands maximal strength and control, and it may take several months of consistent practice to achieve.

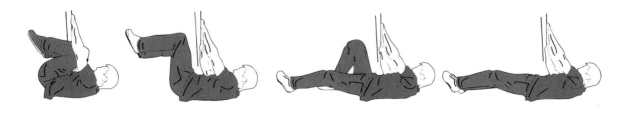

THE NEW CALISTHENICS FORMULA

HOW TO PERFORM THE BACK LEVER

The back lever is another advanced static hold that requires both strength and flexibility. Here's how to approach it:

1. **Skin-the-Cat:** Start by hanging from a bar or rings with your arms straight. Pull your legs through your arms, rotating your body backward until you're upside down, with your feet pointing towards the ground. Continue the rotation until your legs extend behind you, passing through a front lever position. This movement develops the shoulder and core strength needed for the back lever.

2. **Tuck Back Lever:** From the skin-the-cat position, tuck your knees to your chest and lower your body slowly until your back is parallel to the ground. Hold this position, focusing on keeping your core tight and your body aligned. The tuck back lever is less demanding than the full back lever, making it an ideal starting point.

3. **Advanced Tuck Back Lever:** Progress to the advanced tuck by extending your hips while keeping your knees bent. This variation increases the difficulty by shifting more weight away from your center of mass, requiring greater strength and control.

4. **Full Back Lever:** When you're ready, extend your legs fully behind you while maintaining a straight line from your head to your feet. Engage your core and back muscles to hold your body parallel to the ground. Like the front lever, the back lever requires a strong hollow body position to maintain stability and prevent arching in the lower back.

The front lever and back lever are more than just impressive displays of strength—they're a testament to your commitment and progress in calisthenics. By following these progressions and focusing on form, you'll build the strength, stability, and control needed to master these challenging movements. With patience and persistence, you'll be able to hold these positions with confidence and ease, showcasing your hard-earned skills in the world of bodyweight training.

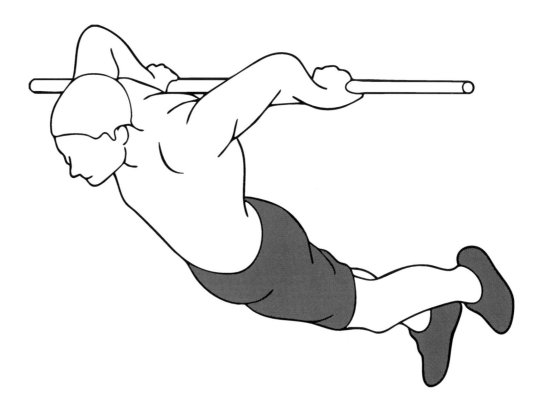

DRAGON FLAGS

Dragon flags are a legendary core exercise that pushes the limits of your abdominal strength and overall body control. Made famous by martial arts icon Bruce Lee, this movement is not only a test of your core but also a full-body challenge that engages your hip flexors, lower back, and even your upper body. The dragon flag requires you to lower and raise your body while maintaining a perfectly straight line, making it one of the most advanced and rewarding exercises in calisthenics.

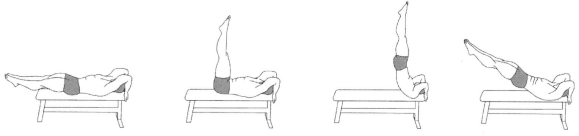

HOW TO PERFORM DRAGON FLAGS

Achieving a full dragon flag requires a step-by-step progression to build the necessary strength and control. Here's how to approach it:

1. **Start with Lying Leg Raises:** Begin by lying flat on your back with your arms extended along your sides or gripping a sturdy object behind your head (like a bench or the legs of a heavy chair). Keep your legs straight and together, and lift them towards the ceiling until they are perpendicular to the ground. Slowly lower your legs back down without letting them touch the ground. Lying leg raises strengthen your lower abs and help you develop the control needed for more advanced movements.

2. **Progress to Hanging Leg Raises:** Hang from a pull-up bar with your arms straight and your legs together. Lift your legs until they are parallel to the ground, focusing on keeping your core tight and your movements controlled. Lower your legs slowly to the starting position. Hanging leg raises increases the difficulty by adding an element of grip strength and lat engagement.

3. **Practice Dragon Flag Negatives:** Once you're comfortable with leg raises, begin practicing the negative phase of the dragon flag. Lie on a bench or flat surface, gripping the edge behind your head with both hands. Lift your legs and hips off the bench, raising your body into a vertical position. Slowly lower your body towards the bench, keeping your legs straight and your core engaged. Focus on maintaining control and keeping your body in a straight line throughout the descent. Dragon flag negatives help you build the strength and stability needed for the full movement.

4. **Full Dragon Flag:** After mastering the negatives, you're ready to attempt the full dragon flag. From the lying position, lift your legs and hips off the bench, bringing your body into a vertical position. Slowly lower your body until it is just above the bench, maintaining a straight line from your shoulders to your feet. Pause briefly at the bottom, then reverse the movement by raising your body back to the starting position. Aim for smooth, controlled execution, avoiding any jerking or bending of your hips.

Dragon flags are more than just a core exercise—they are a full-body challenge that tests your strength, stability, and control. By following a structured progression and focusing on proper form, you'll be able to build the strength needed to execute this iconic movement. With time and dedication, the dragon flag will become a powerful tool in your calisthenics arsenal, helping you achieve a rock-solid core and enhanced overall athleticism.

L-SITS AND V-SITS

L-sits and V-sits are two of the most challenging and rewarding iso-metric exercises in calisthenics. These moves not only build incre-dible core strength but also enhance hip flexor mobility and upper body endurance. The L-sit, with its iconic "L" shape, is a foundational exercise that prepares you for the even more advanced V-sit, where your legs are raised higher to form a "V" shape with your body. Both exercises demand a high level of control, stability, and strength, ma-king them essential skills for anyone serious about calisthenics.

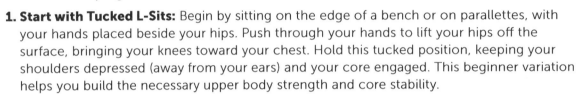

HOW TO PERFORM AN L-SIT

The L-sit is a demanding isometric hold that can be performed on the floor, parallettes, or the edge of a bench. Here's how to progress towards it:

1. **Start with Tucked L-Sits:** Begin by sitting on the edge of a bench or on parallettes, with your hands placed beside your hips. Push through your hands to lift your hips off the surface, bringing your knees toward your chest. Hold this tucked position, keeping your shoulders depressed (away from your ears) and your core engaged. This beginner variation helps you build the necessary upper body strength and core stability.

2. **Extend One Leg at a Time:** Once you're comfortable with the tucked L-sit, begin exten-ding one leg at a time while keeping the other leg tucked. Focus on maintaining straight legs and a strong core with your toes pointed. Alternate between legs to ensure balanced strength development.

3. **Full L-Sit:** When you're ready, extend both legs out in front of you, forming an "L" shape with your body. Keep your legs straight, toes pointed, and core engaged throughout the hold. Aim to hold this position for 10-15 seconds, gradually increasing the duration as you build strength and endurance.

HOW TO PERFORM A V-SIT

The V-sit is an advanced pro-gression from the L-sit, requi-ring greater strength, flexibility, and balance. Here's how to work towards mastering it:

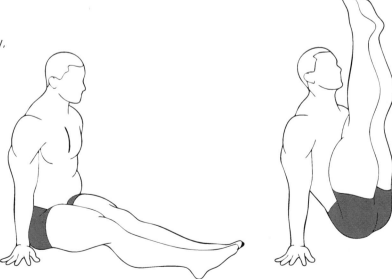

1. **Start with V-Sit Ups:** Lie flat on your back with your arms extended overhead and your legs straight. Simultaneously lift your legs and torso off the ground, aiming to bring your hands toward your feet to form a "V" shape with your body. Lower yourself back down with control and repeat. V-sit ups build the core strength and hip flexor flexibility needed for the V-sit hold.

2. **Work on V-Sit Holds:** Once you can perform V-sit-ups with good form, start practicing the hold position. Sit on the floor or parallettes, with your hands placed beside your hips. Lift your legs and torso to form a "V" shape, balancing on your hands. Focus on keeping your legs straight, toes pointed, and core engaged. Initially, you may only be able to hold this position for a few seconds, but with practice, your strength and endurance will improve.

3. **Gradually Increase the Hold Time:** As your strength and control develop, work on extending the duration of your V-sit hold. Aim for 10-15 seconds initially, and gradually increase the time as you get stronger. Remember to keep your movements smooth and controlled, avoiding any jerking or collapsing of the torso.

Both L-sits and V-sits are powerful additions to any calisthenics routine, offering a challenging way to build core strength, stability, and control. By progressing through these steps and focusing on form, you'll be able to master these isometric holds, showcasing your hard-earned strength and flexibility. With dedication and consistent practice, the L-sit and V-sit will become essential tools in your calisthenics arsenal, helping you achieve a stronger, more resilient body.

MASTERING STATIC HOLDS: ISOMETRIC CHALLENGES

STATIC HOLDS ARE THE ULTIMATE TEST OF STRENGTH, BALANCE, AND MENTAL FOCUS IN CALISTHE-NICS. THEY REQUIRE YOU TO MAINTAIN A POSITION AGAINST THE FORCE OF GRAVITY, OFTEN FOR EXTENDED PERIODS, PUSHING YOUR MUSCLES AND MIND TO THEIR LIMITS. THE HUMAN FLAG, PLAN-CHE, AND OTHER ISOMETRIC CHALLENGES ARE NOT JUST ABOUT STRENGTH; THEY'RE ABOUT CON-TROL AND PRECISION.

HUMAN FLAG

The human flag is one of the most iconic and visually stunning feats in calisthenics, representing a perfect blend of strength, balance, and body control. Holding your body horizontally against a vertical pole, with only your hands gripping the pole for support, is a true testament to the power of your shoulders, lats, and core muscles. Achieving the human flag is no small feat, but with the right progression and dedication, it's an attainable goal.

HOW TO PROGRESS TOWARD THE HUMAN FLAG

Achieving the human flag requires a step-by-step approach, focusing on building the necessary strength and control. Here's how to progress toward this impressive move:

1. **Start with the Vertical Flag:** Begin by gripping a sturdy vertical pole with both hands. Your bottom hand should be in an overhand grip, while your top hand should be in an underhand grip. Position your body vertically, with your feet resting against the pole for support. Focus on engaging your core and lats, and practice holding this position to get comfortable with the grip and body alignment.

2. **Practice the Vertical Flag with Raised Legs:** Once you're comfortable with the basic vertical flag, start lifting your legs higher while maintaining the vertical position. Gradually raise your legs until they are in line with your hips, forming a diagonal line with your body. This progression helps build the shoulder, lat, and core strength needed for the full human flag.

3. **Move to the Assisted Human Flag:** Use a resistance band or have a partner support your legs as you attempt the human flag position. Grip the pole as in the vertical flag, but focus on raising your legs until your body is parallel to the ground. The assistance allows you to work on holding the horizontal position without the full weight of your body, helping you build the strength and control needed for the unassisted flag.

4. **Perform the Tuck Human Flag:** Progress to the tuck human flag, where you tuck your knees towards your chest while holding your body horizontally. This reduces the leverage and makes the position more manageable, allowing you to focus on building strength and stability in the key muscles. Practice holding this position for increasing durations as your strength improves.

5. **Achieve the Full Human Flag:** When you're ready, attempt the full human flag by extending your legs straight out, with your body fully horizontal. Keep your core tight, your lats engaged, and your arms locked out to maintain the position. Start by holding the position for just a few seconds, gradually increasing the duration as you get stronger and more confident.

The human flag is a true test of strength, control, and perseverance. By following these progressions and focusing on building the necessary strength and technique, you can achieve this impressive skill. With time, dedication, and consistent practice, you'll be able to hold the human flag with confidence, showcasing your mastery of one of the most iconic moves in calisthenics.

MALTESE HOLD

The Maltese hold is an advanced static exercise often seen in gymnastics. It involves holding your body parallel to the ground with your arms extended straight out to the sides, supporting your body weight on rings or a bar. This position requires extraordinary strength in the shoulders, chest, and biceps, as well as significant core stability.

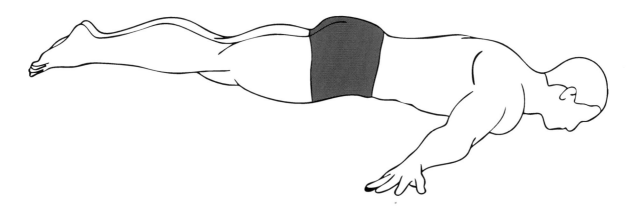

HOW TO PROGRESS TOWARD THE MALTESE HOLD

The Maltese hold is one of the most demanding isometric holds and should be approached with a well-structured progression plan:

1. **Support Hold on Rings:** Start by practicing a support hold on gymnastics rings with your arms fully extended and your body upright. Focus on maintaining a straight arm position and engaging your core and shoulders to stabilize your body. Hold this position for 10-20 seconds, gradually increasing the duration as you build strength.

2. **Tuck Maltese on Rings:** Progress to a tuck Maltese by moving your body forward slightly and tucking your knees into your chest. Your arms should be extended straight out to the sides, supporting your body weight. This position reduces the leverage, allowing you to focus on building the necessary shoulder and chest strength.

3. **Advanced Tuck Maltese:** Once comfortable with the tuck position, extend your hips slightly while keeping your knees bent. This increases the difficulty by shifting more weight onto your arms and requiring greater shoulder stability.

4. **Straddle Maltese:** Move on to the straddle Maltese by extending your legs outward into a straddle position. This position is more challenging but reduces the overall load compared to a full Maltese hold.

5. **Full Maltese Hold:** The final progression is the full Maltese hold, where your body is fully extended and parallel to the ground. Keep your arms straight, and focus on engaging your shoulders, chest, and core to maintain stability. Hold the position for as long as possible, gradually increasing the duration as your strength improves.

The Maltese hold is one of the most challenging static holds in calisthenics and gymnastics, requiring a combination of upper body strength, shoulder stability, and core control. It's a move that demands patience and persistence, but with consistent practice and proper progression, you can develop the strength needed to master this impressive exercise.

IRON CROSS

The Iron Cross is a classic and incredibly challenging static hold primarily seen in gymnastics. It involves holding your body in an upright position on gymnastics rings, with your arms extended straight out to the sides, forming a perfect "T" shape. This exercise requires extraordinary strength in the shoulders, chest, and biceps, as well as impeccable control and stability throughout the entire body.

HOW TO PROGRESS TOWARD THE IRON CROSS

The Iron Cross is one of the most difficult static holds to achieve and demands a well-structured progression plan to build the necessary strength and technique.

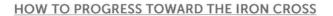

1. **Support Hold on Rings**: Begin by mastering a basic support hold on gymnastics rings. Keep your body upright with your arms extended down by your sides and your core engaged. Focus on maintaining straight arms and a stable position, holding for 10-20 seconds at a time.

2. **Tuck Cross:** From the support position, move your body slightly downwards and outwards, tucking your knees towards your chest. Your arms should be extended outward but at a slightly lower angle than the full Iron Cross. This position reduces leverage, allowing you to build shoulder and chest strength while maintaining control.

3. **Assisted Iron Cross:** Use resistance bands or assistance from a coach or partner to help support your body as you attempt to move into the Iron Cross position. Gradually lower your body into the cross position, keeping your arms straight and using the assistance to maintain stability. Practice holding this position, focusing on engaging your shoulders, chest, and core.

4. **Maltese Cross:** As you gain strength, begin practicing the Maltese Cross, where you hold your body slightly above the Iron Cross position but with your arms fully extended out to the sides. This position is an intermediate step towards the full Iron Cross, helping to build the necessary strength and control.

5. **Full Iron Cross:** When you're ready, attempt the full Iron Cross by lowering your body into the horizontal position with your arms extended straight out to the sides. Focus on keeping your arms straight and your body stable, engaging your shoulders, chest, and biceps to maintain the position. Start by holding the position for just a few seconds, gradually increasing the duration as your strength improves.

The Iron Cross is one of the most demanding and iconic static holds in gymnastics and calisthenics. Achieving this move requires exceptional upper body strength, stability, and control, making it a long-term goal for many athletes. With a disciplined approach to progression and consistent practice, you can develop the strength needed to master the Iron Cross, showcasing your power and precision in one of the most challenging exercises in the world of bodyweight training.

CRAFTING ADVANCED ROUTINES FOR STRENGTH AND SKILL MASTERY

NOW THAT YOU'VE EXPLORED THE ADVANCED EXERCISES AND STATIC HOLDS, IT'S TIME TO CRAFT A ROUTINE THAT WILL HELP YOU MASTER THESE SKILLS. ADVANCED CALISTHENICS TRAINING IS NOT JUST ABOUT DOING MORE REPS OR HOLDING POSITIONS FOR LONGER—IT'S ABOUT SMART PROGRAMMING THAT BALANCES STRENGTH, SKILL WORK, AND RECOVERY.

BALANCING SKILL WORK AND STRENGTH TRAINING

In advanced calisthenics, skill work should be the focus of your training. This means dedicating specific sessions to practicing movements like muscle-ups, planches, and human flags. Start each session with skill practice while your muscles are fresh, and then move on to strength training exercises that complement your skill work.

For example, if you're working on muscle-ups, follow up with weighted pull-ups, dips, and core exercises like L-sits to build the necessary strength. If planches are your focus, include exercises like tuck planche holds, handstand push-ups, and dragon flags in your routine.

INCORPORATING MOBILITY AND FLEXIBILITY

Mobility and flexibility are often overlooked in calisthenics, but they're crucial for preventing injuries and improving performance. Incorporate dynamic stretches and mobility drills into your warm-up and cooldown routines. Focus on areas like your shoulders, hips, and ankles, which are heavily involved in advanced calisthenics movements.

PROGRESSIVE OVERLOAD AND RECOVERY

Just like in weight training, progressive overload is key to making progress in calisthenics. This means gradually increasing the difficulty of your exercises, whether by adding reps, holding positions for longer, or progressing to more challenging variations. Keep track of your progress and adjust your routine accordingly.

Recovery is equally important, especially when training at an advanced level. Make sure to include rest days in your routine and listen to your body. Overtraining can lead to burnout or injury, so prioritize recovery methods like foam rolling, stretching, and adequate sleep to keep your body in top condition.

SAMPLE ADVANCED CALISTHENICS ROUTINE

Here's a sample advanced calisthenics routine that balances skill work, strength training, and recovery:

DAY UPPER BODY SKILL WORK

- **Warm-up:** Dynamic stretches and mobility drills
- **Skill Practice:** Muscle-ups (5 sets of 3-5 reps)

- **Strength Training:** Weighted pull-ups (4 sets of 5-8 reps), Dips (4 sets of 8-10 reps)
- **Core:** L-sits (3 sets of 20-30 seconds), Hanging leg raises (3 sets of 10-12 reps)
- **Cooldown:** Static stretches

DAY  LOWER BODY STRENGTH

- **Warm-up:** Dynamic stretches and mobility drills
- **Strength Training:** Pistol squats (4 sets of 5-8 reps), Shrimp squats (4 sets of 6-10 reps)
- **Plyometrics:** Jumping lunges (3 sets of 10 reps per leg), Box jumps (3 sets of 8-10 reps)
- **Cooldown:** Static stretches

DAY  STATIC HOLDS AND CORE

- **Warm-up:** Dynamic stretches and mobility drills
- **Skill Practice:** Planche progressions (5 sets of 10-15 seconds)
- **Static Holds:** Front lever holds (3 sets of 10-15 seconds), Human flag practice (3 sets of 5-10 seconds)
- **Core:** Dragon flags (3 sets of 5-8 reps), V-sits (3 sets of 15-20 seconds)
- **Cooldown:** Static stretches

DAY  REST AND RECOVERY

- **Active Recovery:** Light cardio (e.g., walking or swimming)
- **Mobility:** Full-body stretching routine
- **Optional:** Foam rolling or massage

DAY FULL BODY SKILL AND STRENGTH

- **Warm-up**: Dynamic stretches and mobility drills
- **Skill Practice:** Handstand push-ups (5 sets of 3-5 reps), Planche holds (5 sets of 10-15 seconds)
- **Strength Training:** Weighted dips (4 sets of 6-8 reps), Shrimp squats (4 sets of 6-10 reps)
- **Core:** L-sits (3 sets of 20-30 seconds), Hanging leg raises (3 sets of 10-12 reps)
- **Cooldown:** Static stretches

DAY ACTIVE REST

- **Active Recovery:** Light cardio or a recreational sport
- **Mobility:** Focused stretching on tight areas

DAY 7 REST AND RECOVERY

- Complete rest day to allow your body to fully recover and prepare for the next week's training

STAYING MOTIVATED ON YOUR ADVANCED CALISTHENICS JOURNEY

Advanced calisthenics requires dedication and patience. Progress may seem slow at times, and the exercises can be frustratingly difficult. But remember, every small improvement is a step closer to mastering your body. Celebrate your milestones, no matter how minor they seem, and keep pushing your limits.

Join a community of like-minded individuals, whether online or in person, to stay motivated and share your journey. Surrounding yourself with others who are also passionate about calisthenics can provide inspiration and support on the days when motivation is low.

Finally, remember that calisthenics is a lifelong journey. There's always a new skill to learn, a new challenge to conquer. Embrace the process, enjoy the journey, and above all, have fun with your training.

Advanced calisthenics mastery is within your reach. With the right mindset, consistent practice, and a well-structured routine, you can unlock new levels of strength, skill, and control over your body. Now, it's time to take action and push your calisthenics journey to new heights.

THE BOTTOM LINE

You've now explored the essentials of advanced calisthenics. From upper and lower body movements to building core strength and tackling challenging static holds, you've seen how each element contributes to your mastery. Crafting routines that push your limits is key to real progress.

As you move forward, the next step is putting it all together. In the upcoming chapter, you'll learn how to structure your calisthenics workout plan for consistent growth and results.

Before you dive in, consider how each advanced move has changed your approach. Which exercises challenge you the most? How will you adapt your routine to keep pushing yourself? Think about where you can refine your technique.

STRUCTURING YOUR CALISTHENICS WORKOUT PLAN

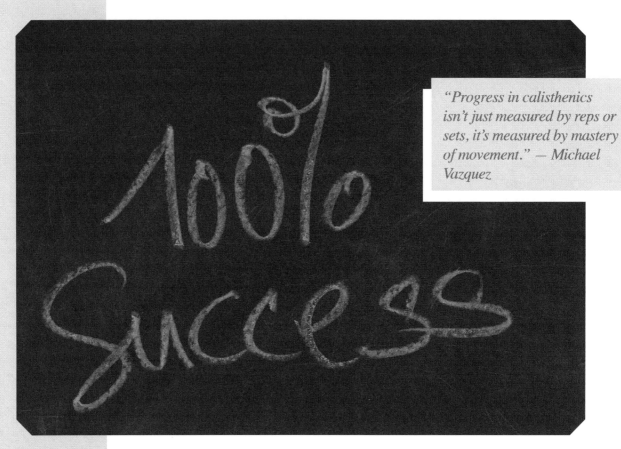

> *"Progress in calisthenics isn't just measured by reps or sets, it's measured by mastery of movement." — Michael Vazquez*

You've decided to embark on a calisthenics journey, a path that promises not only physical strength but also mastery over your own body. But where do you begin? The endless amount of information available can be overwhelming, leaving you unsure of how to start building your workout routine. The good news is that creating a structured calisthenics workout plan doesn't have to be complicated. In fact, by the end of this chapter, you'll have the tools you need to design a workout plan tailored to your unique goals, whether that's building muscle, losing fat, or simply improving your overall fitness. This chapter is your guide to not just understanding the different types of workout plans but also how to personalize them to fit your life and aspirations.

Imagine this: a few months from now, you could be executing flawless muscle-ups, effortlessly flowing from one exercise to the next, your body moving in perfect harmony. Or maybe your goal is to shed some extra pounds, revealing a toned and strong physique beneath. Whatever your goal, the secret lies in structure, consistency, and understanding the mechanics of a well-designed workout plan. So, let's dive in and start building your path to success.

BUILDING YOUR PERSONALIZED WORKOUT ROUTINE

WHEN IT COMES TO CREATING A WORKOUT ROUTINE, ONE SIZE DOES NOT FIT ALL. THE BEAUTY OF CALISTHENICS LIES IN ITS VERSATILITY—YOU CAN TAILOR YOUR WORKOUTS TO FIT YOUR GOALS, WHETHER THAT'S BUILDING STRENGTH, INCREASING MUSCLE MASS, LOSING FAT, OR SIMPLY STAYING ACTIVE AND HEALTHY. BUT BEFORE YOU DIVE INTO THE NITTY-GRITTY, IT'S IMPORTANT TO UNDERSTAND THE BASIC COMPONENTS OF A WELL-ROUNDED WORKOUT PLAN.

UNDERSTANDING THE KEY COMPONENTS

Every effective calisthenics workout plan should include a mix of the following elements:

- **Warm-Up:** This is where you prepare your body for the intense work ahead. A good warm-up increases your heart rate, loosens your joints, and gets your muscles ready for action. Spend at least 5-10 minutes on dynamic stretches or light cardio activities like jumping jacks or running in place.

- **Strength Training:** This is the core of your workout. Strength training in calisthenics involves exercises like push-ups, pull-ups, dips, and squats. These moves challenge your muscles and force them to grow stronger over time.

- **Mobility and Flexibility:** Including exercises that improve your range of motion is crucial. Think of moves like yoga stretches, which help maintain flexibility and prevent injuries.

- **Cool Down:** Just as you need to warm up before a workout, you also need to cool down afterward. This involves stretching and breathing exercises to help your muscles recover and to reduce soreness.

ASSESSING YOUR GOALS AND FITNESS LEVEL

Before you can build your routine, you need to assess where you are and where you want to be. Ask yourself:

- **What is my primary goal?** Are you looking to build strength, gain muscle, lose fat, or improve your overall fitness?

- **What is my current fitness level?** Are you a beginner, intermediate, or advanced athlete? Your current abilities will dictate the intensity and type of exercises you include.

- **How much time can I dedicate to my workouts?** Be realistic about your schedule. Consistency is more important than intensity or duration, especially when you're starting out.

By answering these questions, you're setting the foundation for a workout plan that is not only effective but also sustainable.

CHOOSING YOUR EXERCISES

The exercises you choose should align with your goals. For strength training, focus on compound movements—those that work multiple muscle groups at once. Exercises like push-ups, pull-ups, and squats are staples in any calisthenics routine because they offer a lot of bang for your buck. If flexibility and mobility are more important to you, incorporate yoga poses or dynamic stretches that help improve your range of motion. Here's a simple way to break it down:

- **Upper Body:** Push-ups, pull-ups, dips, and handstand push-ups.

- **Lower Body:** Squats, lunges, pistol squats, and calf raises.

- **Core: Planks,** leg raises, and mountain climbers.

Remember, form is everything. Start with easier variations if necessary, and gradually progress as your strength improves.

STRUCTURING YOUR ROUTINE

Now that you have your goals and exercises in mind, it's time to structure your workout routine. This involves deciding how many days a week you'll train, how to group your exercises, and how much rest you'll need between workouts.

A common approach in calisthenics is to start with a three-day-per-week routine. This allows for sufficient recovery while providing enough frequency to make progress. For example, you might train on Monday, Wednesday, and Friday, giving your muscles time to recover between sessions. Here's a simple template for a full-body workout routine:

DAY 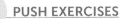 **PUSH EXERCISES**

- Push-ups (3 sets of 10-15 reps)
- Dips (3 sets of 8-12 reps)
- Pike Push-ups (3 sets of 8-12 reps)

DAY **PULL EXERCISES**

- Pull-ups (3 sets of 6-10 reps)
- Inverted Rows (3 sets of 10-15 reps)
- Chin-Ups (3 sets of 12-15 reps)

DAY  **LEG AND CORE EXERCISES**

- Squats (3 sets of 15-20 reps)
- Lunges (3 sets of 10-15 reps per leg)
- Plank (3 sets of 30-60 seconds)

This basic structure covers all major muscle groups and provides a solid foundation for further progression. As you advance, you can add more exercises, increase the number of sets, or experiment with different variations.

FULL-BODY VS. SPLIT ROUTINES: WHICH IS RIGHT FOR YOU?

ONE OF THE BIGGEST DECISIONS YOU'LL NEED TO MAKE WHEN STRUCTURING YOUR CALISTHENICS WORKOUT PLAN IS WHETHER TO FOCUS ON FULL-BODY WORKOUTS OR SPLIT ROUTINES. BOTH APPROACHES HAVE THEIR BENEFITS AND DRAWBACKS, AND THE RIGHT CHOICE DEPENDS LARGELY ON YOUR GOALS, SCHEDULE, AND PERSONAL PREFERENCE.

FULL-BODY WORKOUTS

Full-body workouts involve exercising all major muscle groups in a single session. This approach is particularly effective if you're short on time or if you're a beginner just getting started with calisthenics. By hitting every muscle group, you ensure balanced development and can maximize your workout time.

BENEFITS OF FULL-BODY WORKOUTS

- **Efficiency:** You train all major muscle groups in one session, which is great if you can only work out a few times a week.

- **Increased Caloric Burn:** Full-body workouts tend to burn more calories because they involve more muscles and movement.

- **Balanced Development:** By working your entire body, you avoid the risk of muscle imbalances.

DRAWBACKS

- **Longer Recovery Time:** Because you're working out your entire body, you may need more time to recover between sessions.

- **Fatigue:** Training all major muscle groups in one session can be exhausting, which might affect your performance on later exercises.

SPLIT ROUTINES

Split routines involve focusing on specific muscle groups on different days. For example, you might do upper body exercises one day and lower body exercises the next. This approach is often preferred by those who have more time to dedicate to their workouts and want to focus on building strength or muscle mass in specific areas.

BENEFITS OF SPLIT ROUTINES

- **Targeted Training:** Allows you to focus more intensely on specific muscle groups, which can lead to greater strength or hypertrophy in those areas.

- **Shorter Sessions:** Each workout is generally shorter because you're focusing on fewer exercises.

- **Better Recovery:** Since you're not working the same muscle groups every day, your muscles have more time to recover.

- **Time Commitment:** Split routines typically require more days of training per week.

- **Risk of Imbalance:** If not carefully planned, split routines can lead to muscle imbalances if certain areas are neglected.

CHOOSING THE RIGHT ROUTINE FOR YOU

So, which routine is right for you? The answer depends on your goals, experience level, and time availability. If you're a beginner or have a tight schedule, full-body workouts might be the best way to start. They're efficient, easy to structure, and provide a solid foundation. As you progress and if your goals become more specific—such as building muscle in a particular area—you might consider transitioning to a split routine.

Here's a practical tip: Start with a full-body routine and assess your progress after 4-6 weeks. If you feel that certain areas need more attention, gradually introduce split routines into your plan. The key is to listen to your body and adjust as needed.

It's also worth noting that you don't have to stick to one approach forever. Many athletes find success by alternating between full-body and split routines, depending on their current goals and how their body is responding to training. The key is to listen to your body and adjust your routine as needed to continue making progress.

SCHEDULING REST AND RECOVERY FOR OPTIMAL PERFORMANCE

IT'S TEMPTING TO THINK THAT THE MORE YOU TRAIN, THE FASTER YOU'LL SEE RESULTS. HOWEVER, RECOVERY IS WHERE THE MAGIC HAPPENS. IT'S DURING THIS TIME THAT YOUR MUSCLES REPAIR AND GROW, YOUR NERVOUS SYSTEM ADAPTS, AND YOUR BODY BECOMES STRONGER. WITHOUT ADEQUATE RECOVERY, YOU RISK OVERTRAINING, WHICH CAN LEAD TO INJURIES, BURNOUT, AND EVEN REGRESSION IN YOUR PROGRESS. THIS IS WHY IT'S ESSENTIAL TO INCORPORATE REST DAYS INTO YOUR WORKOUT PLAN AND PAY ATTENTION TO YOUR BODY'S SIGNALS.

THE IMPORTANCE OF RECOVERY

Recovery isn't just about taking a day off; it's an active part of your training plan. When you work out, you're essentially breaking down muscle fibers. It's during recovery that these fibers rebuild and become stronger. Skipping rest days or not allowing your body enough time to recover can lead to overtraining—a condition that not only hampers progress but can also lead to serious injuries. Here's what you need to know about scheduling rest:

- **Active Recovery:** This involves light activities like walking, stretching, or yoga. It keeps your body moving without putting too much strain on your muscles. Active recovery days are great for maintaining flexibility and promoting blood flow to sore muscles.

- **Rest Days:** Complete rest days are crucial, especially if you're doing intense training. On these days, avoid strenuous activities and focus on relaxation. Think of it as recharging your battery.

- **Sleep:** Never underestimate the power of a good night's sleep. It's during sleep that your body does most of its repair work. Aim for at least 7-9 hours of quality sleep per night.

HOW TO SCHEDULE YOUR REST DAYS

The number of rest days you need depends on your workout intensity, volume, and personal recovery rate. As a general rule:

- **Beginners:** Start with 2-3 rest days per week. This gives your body ample time to adapt to your new routine.

- **Intermediate:** As you build strength, you might reduce rest days to 1-2 per week, incorporating active recovery on lighter days.

- **Advanced:** If you're training at a high intensity, consider having at least one full rest day and one active recovery day each week.

SIGNS YOU NEED MORE REST

It's important to listen to your body. If you experience any of the following, it might be time to take an extra rest day:

- Persistent muscle soreness
- Decreased performance
- Fatigue or irritability
- Trouble sleeping
- Increased heart rate at rest

Remember, it's better to rest and recover than to push through and risk injury. Think of rest as an investment in your long-term fitness success.

WORKOUT PLAN EXAMPLES FOR DIFFERENT GOALS

NOT ALL WORKOUT PLANS ARE CREATED EQUAL. DEPENDING ON WHETHER YOUR GOAL IS TO BUILD STRENGTH, GAIN MUSCLE, LOSE FAT, OR IMPROVE OVERALL FITNESS, THE STRUCTURE OF YOUR CALISTHENICS ROUTINE WILL VARY. BELOW, WE'LL BREAK DOWN SAMPLE WORKOUT PLANS FOR DIFFERENT GOALS, BUT REMEMBER, THESE ARE JUST TEMPLATES. FEEL FREE TO TWEAK THEM BASED ON YOUR PERSONAL PREFERENCES AND PROGRESS.

STRENGTH BUILDING

If your goal is to build strength, your focus should be on low-rep, high-intensity exercises. Strength training in calisthenics involves challenging your muscles with exercises that require maximum effort for a few repetitions.

SAMPLE STRENGTH-BUILDING ROUTINE

DAY FULL BODY

- Push-Ups: 4 sets of 6-8 reps
- Pull-Ups: 4 sets of 4-6 reps
- Pistol Squats: 4 sets of 5 reps per leg
- Dips: 3 sets of 6-8 reps
- Plank: 3 sets of 60 seconds

DAY ACTIVE RECOVERY

- Light Jogging (20-30 minutes)
- Stretching or Yoga (30 minutes)

DAY UPPER BODY FOCUS

- Handstand Push-Ups: 4 sets of 4-6 reps
- Chin-Ups: 4 sets of 4-6 reps
- Archer Push-Ups: 3 sets of 5 reps per side
- L-Sit: 3 sets of 30 seconds

DAY LOWER BODY FOCUS

- Bulgarian Split Squats: 4 sets of 6 reps per leg
- Single-Leg Calf Raises: 3 sets of 10 reps per leg
- Box Jumps: 3 sets of 8 reps
- Glute Bridges: 3 sets of 10 reps

DAY REST OR ACTIVE RECOVERY

- Day 6: Full Body
- Muscle-Ups: 3 sets of 3-5 reps
- Deep Dips: 4 sets of 5-7 reps
- Explosive Push-Ups: 4 sets of 8 reps
- Hanging Leg Raises: 3 sets of 8 reps

DAY REST

Strength-building routines focus on low reps with high intensity. Each exercise is carefully chosen to target multiple muscle groups, ensuring balanced strength development.

MUSCLE GAIN (HYPERTROPHY)

When it comes to building muscle, also known as hypertrophy, the key is to focus on moderate reps with controlled form. The goal is to create muscle tension over a longer period, which stimulates muscle growth.

SAMPLE MUSCLE GAIN ROUTINE

DAY **PUSH DAY (UPPER BODY)**

• Push-Ups: 4 sets of 8-12 reps
• Dips: 4 sets of 8-12 reps
• Diamond Push-Ups: 3 sets of 10-12 reps
• Triceps Extensions: 3 sets of 10-15 reps

DAY **PULL DAY (UPPER BODY)**

• Pull-Ups: 4 sets of 8-10 reps
• Australian Pull-Ups: 3 sets of 12-15 reps
• Chin-Ups: 3 sets of 8-10 reps
• Bicep Curls (using bands): 3 sets of 12-15 reps

DAY **LEG DAY**

• Squats: 4 sets of 12-15 reps
• Lunges: 3 sets of 12 reps per leg
• Calf Raises: 3 sets of 15 reps
• Glute Bridges: 3 sets of 12-15 reps

DAY **REST OR ACTIVE RECOVERY**

DAY **CORE AND STABILITY**

• Plank: 3 sets of 60 seconds
• Hanging Leg Raises: 4 sets of 8-10 reps
• Side Plank: 3 sets of 45 seconds per side
• Mountain Climbers: 3 sets of 15 reps per leg

DAY **FULL BODY CIRCUIT**

• Circuit 1: Push-Ups, Squats, Pull-Ups (3 rounds, 10-12 reps each)
• Circuit 2: Dips, Lunges, Plank (3 rounds, 10-12 reps each)
• Circuit 3: Handstand Hold, Bulgarian Split Squats, Bicycle Crunches (3 rounds, 10-12 reps each)

DAY **REST**

Hypertrophy routines focus on moderate reps with consistent tension. The use of circuits and targeted exercises promotes muscle growth across different areas.

FAT LOSS AND TONING

If your goal is to lose fat and tone up, your workout plan should include high-rep exercises and cardio-based movements. The aim is to keep your heart rate elevated while building lean muscle.

SAMPLE FAT LOSS AND TONING ROUTINE

DAY **FULL BODY HIIT**

- Jump Squats: 4 sets of 15 reps
- Push-Ups: 4 sets of 15 reps
- Burpees: 3 sets of 12 reps
- High Knees: 3 sets of 30 seconds
- Mountain Climbers: 3 sets of 15 reps per leg

DAY **ACTIVE RECOVERY**

- Light Jogging (20-30 minutes)
- Stretching or Yoga (30 minutes)

DAY **UPPER BODY BURN**

- Push-Ups: 4 sets of 15 reps
- Pull-Ups: 4 sets of 8-10 reps
- Dips: 4 sets of 12 reps
- Plank: 3 sets of 60 seconds

DAY **LOWER BODY BURN**

- Squats: 4 sets of 15 reps
- Lunges: 4 sets of 12 reps per leg
- Box Jumps: 3 sets of 15 reps
- Jump Rope: 3 sets of 60 seconds

DAY **FULL BODY CIRCUIT**

- Circuit 1: Push-Ups, Squats, Plank (3 rounds, 15 reps each)
- Circuit 2: Dips, Lunges, High Knees (3 rounds, 15 reps each)
- Circuit 3: Burpees, Jump Squats, Mountain Climbers (3 rounds, 15 reps each)

DAY **REST OR ACTIVE RECOVERY**

DAY **CARDIO DAY**

30-45 minutes of running, cycling, or swimming
Fat loss routines emphasize calorie burn through high reps and continuous movement. The mix of strength and cardio helps tone muscles while shedding excess fat.

HOW TO ADJUST YOUR WORKOUT PLAN OVER TIME

AS YOU PROGRESS IN YOUR CALISTHENICS JOURNEY, YOUR WORKOUT PLAN SHOULD EVOLVE. STICKING TO THE SAME ROUTINE FOR TOO LONG CAN LEAD TO PLATEAUS, WHERE YOUR PROGRESS STALLS, AND YOUR BODY NO LONGER RESPONDS TO THE EXERCISES. ADJUSTING YOUR PLAN OVER TIME IS CRUCIAL FOR CONTINUED SUCCESS AND REACHING YOUR FITNESS GOALS.

MONITORING YOUR PROGRESS

As you follow your workout plan, it's important to regularly assess your progress. This could involve tracking your strength gains, measuring your body composition, or simply noting how you feel during and after your workouts. Monitoring your progress allows you to see how your body is responding to your routine and identify areas where you might need to make adjustments.

WHEN TO MAKE CHANGES

There are several signs that it might be time to adjust your workout plan. If you've been following the same routine for several weeks and notice that your progress has stalled, it could be a sign that your body has adapted to the exercises. In this case, you might need to increase the intensity of your workouts, either by adding more reps, sets, or weight (if you're using equipment) or by progressing to more advanced exercises.

Another reason to adjust your plan is if you're experiencing any signs of overtraining, such as persistent fatigue, irritability, or a lack of motivation to train. In this case, you might need to incorporate more rest days or switch to a less intense routine temporarily.

PROGRESSIVE OVERLOAD: THE KEY TO CONTINUOUS IMPROVEMENT

One of the most effective ways to ensure you keep progressing is by applying the principle of progressive overload. This means gradually increasing the intensity of your workouts by adding more reps, sets, or resistance or by performing more challenging exercise variations.

For example:

• If you can easily perform ten push-ups, try increasing to 12 or 15.
• Add a weighted vest or resistance bands to your bodyweight exercises.
• Progress from standard push-ups to more advanced variations like diamond push-ups or archer push-ups.

PERIODIZATION: STRUCTURING YOUR TRAINING CYCLES

Periodization involves organizing your training into cycles, each with a specific focus. This approach helps prevent burnout and overtraining while promoting consistent progress. A typical periodization model includes phases like:

• Hypertrophy (Muscle Building) Phase: Focus on moderate reps and volume to build muscle mass.
• Strength Phase: Lower reps, higher intensity to build raw strength.
• Endurance Phase: Higher reps, lower intensity to improve muscular endurance.
• Rest and Recovery Phase: Incorporate de-load weeks or active recovery to allow your body to fully recover.

By cycling through these phases every few months, you can keep your workouts fresh and your body continually adapting.

LISTEN TO YOUR BODY

Adjusting your workout plan isn't just about adding more reps or changing exercises. It's also about listening to your body and responding to its needs. Some days, you might feel strong and capable of pushing yourself harder; other days, you might need to back off and focus on lighter work or recovery.

Being in tune with your body's signals is a skill that develops over time. It's okay to modify your plan based on how you're feeling—this kind of flexibility is key to long-term success.

THE BOTTOM LINE

Building a calisthenics workout plan is not just about choosing the right exercises or sticking to a schedule—it's about understanding your body, setting clear goals, and staying committed to the process. As you progress, remember that the journey is just as important as the destination. Every rep, every set, and every drop of sweat is a step closer to becoming the best version of yourself.

Whether your goal is to build strength, gain muscle, lose fat, or simply improve your overall fitness, this chapter has provided you with the tools to create a workout plan that's tailored to your unique needs. Now, it's up to you to put in the work, stay consistent, and watch as your body transforms through the power of calisthenics. So, are you ready to take the next step in your fitness journey? The plan is in your hands—now it's time to make it happen.

CALISTHENICS FOR FAT LOSS AND LEAN MUSCLE BUILDING

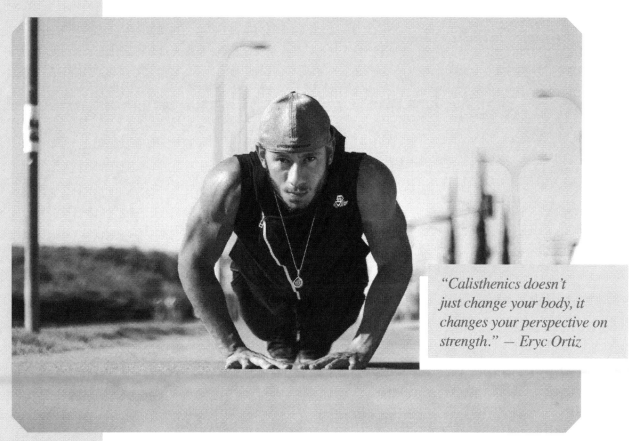

"Calisthenics doesn't just change your body, it changes your perspective on strength." — Eryc Ortiz

Have you ever wondered how you can burn fat and build lean muscle without setting foot in a gym? The answer lies in calisthenics, a form of bodyweight training that not only sculpts your physique but also melts fat efficiently. Whether you're a fitness enthusiast or just starting on your journey, calisthenics offers a holistic approach to fat loss and muscle building. By utilizing nothing more than your body weight, you can achieve the kind of physique that people typically associate with weightlifting or hours of cardio. The beauty of calisthenics is its simplicity and accessibility—you don't need fancy equipment, just your own body and determination.

In this chapter, we will explore how calisthenics works for fat loss and lean muscle building, focusing on high-intensity interval training (HIIT) and metabolic conditioning circuits. You'll also get practical, fat-burning workouts that help maintain muscle, ensuring you see progress without sacrificing strength.

HOW CALISTHENICS HELPS BURN FAT AND BUILD LEAN MUSCLE

YOU MIGHT BE WONDERING, "CAN SIMPLE BODYWEIGHT EXERCISES REALLY HELP ME LOSE FAT AND BUILD MUSCLE?" THE ANSWER IS A RESOUNDING YES. CALISTHENICS, AT ITS CORE, IS ABOUT HARNESSING THE POWER OF YOUR OWN BODY WEIGHT TO CREATE RESISTANCE. THE EXERCISES YOU PERFORM, SUCH AS PUSH-UPS, SQUATS, AND PULL-UPS, ENGAGE MULTIPLE MUSCLE GROUPS AT ONCE. THIS FULL-BODY ENGAGEMENT INCREASES YOUR HEART RATE AND FORCES YOUR MUSCLES TO WORK HARDER THAN THEY WOULD WITH ISOLATED WEIGHT TRAINING. IT'S THIS CONSTANT, DYNAMIC MOVEMENT THAT ACCELERATES FAT LOSS WHILE PROMOTING LEAN MUSCLE DEVELOPMENT.

CALISTHENICS: A NATURAL FAT BURNER

When you perform calisthenics, you're engaging your muscles in compound movements, which means that multiple joints and muscle groups are working together. This burns more calories than isolated exercises and, over time, helps reduce body fat. The key is consistency and progression. The more you challenge your muscles, the more calories you burn, even after your workout is over—thanks to a phenomenon called excess post-exercise oxygen consumption (EPOC). EPOC means your body continues to burn calories as it works to restore itself to its pre-exercise state.

For example, exercises like burpees and mountain climbers are excellent fat burners because they combine cardio and strength, pushing your heart rate up while toning your muscles. In one study, researchers found that high-intensity calisthenics led to significant fat loss in participants over a 12-week period, especially around the abdomen, where fat is often most stubborn.

BUILDING LEAN MUSCLE WITH CALISTHENICS

Lean muscle is the foundation of a toned, sculpted body. Unlike bulky muscle mass, lean muscle gives you strength and endurance without excessive size. Calisthenics excels in building lean muscle because it emphasizes functional strength—the kind you use in everyday activities. Every time you perform a push-up or a squat, you're not just isolating one muscle; you're training your body to work as a cohesive unit, which leads to more balanced muscle development.

A great example of this is the pull-up. It may seem like an arm exercise, but it engages your entire upper body, including your back, shoulders, and core. Over time, pull-ups will help you build a strong, lean upper body that supports fat loss because muscle burns more calories than fat, even when you're resting.

HIGH-INTENSITY INTERVAL TRAINING (HIIT) WITH CALISTHENICS

IF YOU'RE LOOKING TO SUPERCHARGE YOUR FAT-BURNING AND MUSCLE-BUILDING EFFORTS, INCORPORATING HIGH-INTENSITY INTERVAL TRAINING (HIIT) INTO YOUR CALISTHENICS ROUTINE IS THE WAY TO GO. THE CONCEPT BEHIND HIIT IS SIMPLE: YOU PERFORM EXERCISES AT A HIGH INTENSITY FOR A SHORT PERIOD, FOLLOWED BY A BRIEF REST OR LOW-INTENSITY PERIOD. THIS ALTERNATION BETWEEN HIGH AND LOW INTENSITY KEEPS YOUR HEART RATE ELEVATED, TURNING YOUR BODY INTO A FAT-BURNING MACHINE.

WHY HIIT WORKS

HIIT works so well for fat loss because it spikes your heart rate quickly, increasing calorie burn during and after your workout. A study published in the Journal of Obesity highlighted that participants who performed HIIT workouts experienced a significant reduction in body fat compared to those who did steady-state cardio.

With calisthenics, you can perform HIIT circuits without needing any equipment. For instance, you can do 30 seconds of high-intensity squats, followed by 15 seconds of rest, then jump into 30 seconds of push-ups, and so on. The key is to push yourself during those 30 seconds—maximizing the intensity to get the most out of your workout.

BENEFITS OF HIIT WITH CALISTHENICS

- **Increased Fat Burn:** HIIT keeps your metabolism elevated long after the workout ends.

- **Improved Cardiovascular Health:** The constant spikes in heart rate improve heart function and endurance.

- **Muscle Preservation:** Unlike steady-state cardio, HIIT allows you to maintain and even build muscle while shedding fat.

- **Time Efficiency:** HIIT workouts can be done in 20-30 minutes, making them perfect for busy schedules.

INTEGRATING CALISTHENICS INTO HIIT

Combining calisthenics with HIIT creates a potent workout regimen that builds strength, endurance, and accelerates fat loss simultaneously. Here's how you can blend these two powerful training methods effectively.

SELECTING THE RIGHT EXERCISES

Choose exercises that engage multiple muscle groups and can be performed at high intensity. Some excellent calisthenics exercises for HIIT include:

- Burpees: A full-body movement that boosts heart rate and builds strength.
- Jump Squats: Targets the lower body while adding a cardiovascular element.
- Mountain Climbers: Engages the core and improves agility.
- Push-Ups: Builds upper body strength and can be intensified by increasing speed.
- High Knees: Elevates heart rate and works the legs and core.

A typical HIIT session involves short bursts of intense activity followed by brief rest periods. For example:

- 20 seconds of maximum-effort burpees
- 10-second rest
- 20 seconds of jump squats
- 10-second rest
- Continue this pattern with different exercises for a total of 15-20 minutes.

This format, known as the Tabata protocol, is highly effective and time-efficient.

SAMPLE HIIT CALISTHENICS ROUTINE

Here's a sample routine you can try:

WARM-UP (5 MINUTES):

- Light jogging in place
- Arm circles
- Bodyweight squats
- Lunges
- Dynamic stretches

WORKOUT (20 MINUTES):

Perform each exercise for 30 seconds at maximum intensity, followed by 15 seconds of rest. Repeat the entire circuit four times.

1. Jumping Jacks
2. Push-Ups
3. High Knees
4. Mountain Climbers
5. Squat Jumps
6. Plank Hold

COOL-DOWN (5 MINUTES):

- Slow walking
- Static stretches focusing on major muscle groups
- Deep breathing exercises

TIPS FOR EFFECTIVE HIIT CALISTHENICS TRAINING

- **Maintain Proper Form**: Even at high intensity, prioritize correct form to prevent injuries and ensure maximum effectiveness.

- **Listen to Your Body:** Push yourself but know your limits. It's okay to modify exercises or take longer rest periods as needed.

- **Stay Consistent:** Aim for 2-3 HIIT sessions per week, allowing adequate rest and recovery between workouts.
- **Stay Hydrated:** Drink plenty of water before, during, and after your workouts to stay hydrated and aid recovery.

METABOLIC CONDITIONING AND FAT-BURNING CIRCUITS

TAKING YOUR FITNESS JOURNEY A STEP FURTHER, LET'S EXPLORE METABOLIC CONDITIONING— ANOTHER POWERFUL APPROACH THAT UTILIZES CALISTHENICS TO OPTIMIZE FAT LOSS AND ENHANCE OVERALL ATHLETIC PERFORMANCE.

WHAT IS METABOLIC CONDITIONING?

Metabolic conditioning, often referred to as "metcon," involves structured patterns of work and rest periods designed to maximize the efficiency of your body's energy systems. These workouts are typically high-intensity and incorporate compound movements that challenge multiple muscle groups, elevating your heart rate and accelerating calorie burn.

THE THREE ENERGY SYSTEMS

Understanding metabolic conditioning involves grasping how your body's energy systems work:

1. **Phosphagen System:** Provides immediate energy for short, explosive movements (e.g., sprints, jumps).
2. **Glycolytic System:** Supplies energy for moderate-duration, high-intensity activities.
3. **Oxidative System:** Fuels longer-duration, lower-intensity activities.

Metcon workouts strategically tax these systems to improve your body's ability to generate and utilize energy efficiently, leading to enhanced endurance, strength, and fat loss.

IMPLEMENTING CALISTHENICS IN METABOLIC CONDITIONING

Calisthenics exercises are ideal for metcon workouts due to their versatility and ability to engage various muscle groups effectively. Here's how to structure a calisthenics-based metabolic conditioning routine.

CHOOSING EFFECTIVE EXERCISES

Select a mix of exercises that target different parts of the body and vary in intensity and complexity. Examples include:

- Pull-Ups: Strengthens the back and biceps.
- Pistol Squats: Challenges leg strength and balance.
- Handstand Push-Ups: Develops shoulder and core strength.
- Box Jumps: Enhances explosive power and leg strength.
- Dips: Targets the chest, shoulders, and triceps.

THE NEW CALISTHENICS FORMULA

A typical metcon circuit involves performing a series of exercises back-to-back with minimal rest, followed by a designated rest period before repeating the circuit. For example:

Circuit Structure:

• Pull-Ups: 10 reps
• Pistol Squats: 10 reps each leg
• Handstand Push-Ups: 8 reps
• Box Jumps: 12 reps
• Dips: 15 reps

Rest: 2 minutes

Repeat: 3-4 rounds

This structure keeps your heart rate elevated and muscles engaged, promoting significant calorie burn and metabolic boost.

BENEFITS OF METABOLIC CONDITIONING

• **Increased Fat Loss:** By keeping your heart rate elevated, MetCon circuits help you burn more calories in less time.

• **Enhanced Muscle Definition:** The variety of exercises targets multiple muscle groups, ensuring balanced development.

• **Better Endurance:** MetCon circuits improve both muscular and cardiovascular endurance.

SAMPLE METABOLIC CONDITIONING CIRCUIT

WARM-UP (5 MINUTES):

• Jump rope
• Dynamic stretches focusing on major muscle groups
• Light jogging

WORKOUT (25 MINUTES):

Perform each exercise sequentially with minimal rest. After completing all exercises, rest for 2 minutes and repeat the circuit 3 times.

1. **Burpees**: 12 reps
2. **Pull-Ups**: 10 reps
3. **Walking Lunges**: 20 reps (10 each leg)
4. **Push-Ups**: 15 reps
5. **Jump Squats**: 12 reps
6. **Plank Hold**: 60 seconds

<u>COOL-DOWN (5 MINUTES):</u>

- Slow walking to lower heart rate
- Static stretches targeting worked muscles
- Deep breathing exercises

NUTRITION AND RECOVERY CONSIDERATIONS

To maximize the benefits of metabolic conditioning, pay attention to your nutrition and recovery:

- **Balanced Diet:** Fuel your body with a mix of proteins, carbohydrates, and healthy fats to support energy needs and muscle repair.

- **Stay Hydrated:** Adequate hydration is crucial for performance and recovery.

- **Adequate Rest**: Ensure you get enough sleep and rest days to allow your body to recover and prevent overtraining.

- **Listen to Your Body:** Modify workouts as needed based on your fitness level and how your body responds.

SAMPLE FAT-LOSS FOCUSED WORKOUTS

NOW THAT WE'VE EXPLORED THE PRINCIPLES BEHIND USING CALISTHENICS FOR FAT LOSS AND MUSCLE BUILDING LET'S LOOK AT SOME PRACTICAL, READY-TO-USE WORKOUTS YOU CAN INCORPORATE INTO YOUR ROUTINE. THESE WORKOUTS ARE DESIGNED TO BE FLEXIBLE AND ADAPTABLE TO VARIOUS FITNESS LEVELS.

WORKOUT 1: FULL-BODY FAT BLASTER

<u>DURATION: 30 MINUTES</u>

Perform each exercise for the specified number of reps or time, with 30 seconds of rest between exercises. Complete three rounds of the circuit with 2 minutes rest between rounds.

Exercises:

1. **Jumping Jacks**: 50 reps
2. **Push-Ups:** 15 reps (modify to knee push-ups if needed)
3. **Walking Lunges:** 20 reps (10 each leg)
4. **Mountain Climbers:** 40 reps (20 each leg)
5. **Squat Jumps:** 15 reps
6. **Plank:** 60 seconds
7. **Burpees:** 10 reps

Instructions:

- Warm-up: Start with 5 minutes of light cardio and dynamic stretches.

- Execution: Maintain proper form throughout each exercise. Adjust rest periods as needed based on your fitness level.

- Cool-down: Finish with 5 minutes of static stretching, focusing on all major muscle groups.

WORKOUT 2: UPPER BODY AND CORE FOCUS

DURATION: 25 MINUTES

Perform each exercise for 45 seconds, followed by 15-second rest. Complete 4 rounds with 1-minute rest between rounds.

Exercises:

1. Pull-Ups or Inverted Rows (use a sturdy table or bar): 45 seconds
2. Push-Ups: 45 seconds
3. Dips (using parallel bars or a sturdy chair): 45 seconds
4. Russian Twists: 45 seconds
5. Hollow Body Hold: 45 seconds

Instructions:

- Warm-up: 5 minutes of light cardio and dynamic upper body stretches.
- Execution: Focus on controlled movements and engaging the targeted muscle groups effectively.
- Cool-down: 5 minutes of stretching, emphasizing the chest, back, shoulders, and core.

WORKOUT 3: LOWER BODY AND CARDIO BURN

DURATION: 30 MINUTES

Perform each exercise for 30 seconds with a 15-second rest. Complete 5 rounds with 2 minutes rest between rounds.

Exercises:

1. **High Knees**
2. **Bodyweight Squats**
3. **Alternating Reverse Lunges**
4. **Glute Bridges**
5. **Lateral Bounds (side-to-side jumps)**
6. **Calf Raises**

Instructions:

- Warm-up: 5 minutes of brisk walking or jogging and dynamic lower body stretches.
- Execution: Keep movements controlled and focus on engaging the muscles effectively, increasing speed during cardio-focused exercises for added intensity.
- Cool-down: 5 minutes of stretching focusing on the legs, hips, and lower back.

WORKOUT 4: HIIT CALISTHENICS CHALLENGE

DURATION: 20 MINUTES

20 seconds of maximum effort followed by a 10-second rest (Tabata protocol). Complete 8 rounds of each exercise before moving to the next, with 1-minute rest between exercises.

Exercises:

1. **Burpees**
2. **Jump Squats**
3. **Push-Ups**
4. **Mountain Climbers**

Instructions:

- Warm-up: 5 minutes of light cardio and full-body dynamic stretches.

- Execution: Push yourself during the work periods while maintaining good form. Use rest periods to catch your breath and prepare for the next interval.

- Cool-down: 5 minutes of slow walking and full-body stretching.

WORKOUT 5: METABOLIC CONDITIONING CIRCUIT

DURATION: 35 MINUTES

Perform each exercise for the specified reps, moving from one to the next with minimal rest. Complete three rounds with three minutes of rest between rounds.

Exercises:

1. **Pull-Ups:** 8 reps
2. **Plyometric Push-Ups (clap push-ups or explosive push-ups):** 10 reps
3. **Pistol Squats:** 6 reps each leg
4. **Burpees:** 12 reps
5. **Walking Lunges with Knee Raise:** 10 reps on each leg
6. **V-Ups:** 15 reps
7. **Box Jumps:** 10 reps

Instructions:

- Warm-up: 5-7 minutes of light cardio and dynamic stretches targeting all major muscle groups.

- Execution: Focus on explosive movements where applicable and maintain proper form to maximize benefits and prevent injury.

- Cool-down: 5-7 minutes of static stretching and deep breathing exercises.

CUSTOMIZING WORKOUTS TO YOUR FITNESS LEVEL

Remember, these workouts are templates and can be adjusted to suit your current fitness level:

BEGINNER MODIFICATIONS:

Reduce the number of rounds or reps.
Increase rest periods between exercises and rounds.
Modify exercises (e.g., knee push-ups instead of standard push-ups).

ADVANCED ENHANCEMENTS:

Increase the intensity by adding more reps or rounds.
Decrease rest periods.
Incorporate more challenging variations of exercises (e.g., one-arm push-ups).

HOW TO MAINTAIN MUSCLE WHILE LOSING FAT

ACHIEVING FAT LOSS WHILE PRESERVING, OR EVEN BUILDING, MUSCLE MASS IS A DELICATE BALANCE THAT REQUIRES STRATEGIC PLANNING IN BOTH YOUR TRAINING AND NUTRITION. LET'S EXPLORE EFFECTIVE STRATEGIES TO HELP YOU MAINTAIN YOUR HARD-EARNED MUSCLE WHILE SHEDDING EXCESS FAT.

PRIORITIZE PROTEIN IN YOUR DIET

To maintain muscle, you must prioritize protein in your diet. Protein supports muscle repair and growth, especially when you're in a calorie deficit. Aim for about 1.6 to 2.2 grams of protein per kilogram of body weight per day, as recommended by several studies on muscle preservation during fat loss.

INCLUDE STRENGTH-BASED CALISTHENICS

To preserve muscle, include strength-based calisthenics exercises such as push-ups, pull-ups, and dips in your routine. These exercises target your major muscle groups and promote muscle retention, even while you're burning fat. Additionally, exercises like the planche and handstand push-ups challenge your muscles in new ways, ensuring continued strength gains.

AVOID EXTREME CALORIE DEFICITS

While it might be tempting to cut calories drastically, doing so can lead to muscle loss. Instead, aim for a moderate calorie deficit that allows you to lose 0.5 to 1 kg of fat per week while preserving lean muscle.

REST AND RECOVERY

Your muscles need time to recover and grow. Make sure you get enough rest between workouts and prioritize sleep. Studies have shown that inadequate sleep can hinder fat loss and lead to muscle loss.

THE BOTTOM LINE

Calisthenics offers a natural, accessible way to burn fat and build lean muscle, making it a powerful tool for anyone looking to improve their fitness. Whether through HIIT, metabolic conditioning, or strength-based circuits, these exercises push your body to work harder, torching calories while building functional strength.

By incorporating the strategies and workouts outlined in this chapter, you can achieve a lean, strong physique without the need for a gym or heavy weights. Remember, consistency is key—stick to your routine, fuel your body with the right nutrients, and watch as your body transforms, becoming stronger, leaner, and healthier every day.

RECOVERY AND INJURY PREVENTION

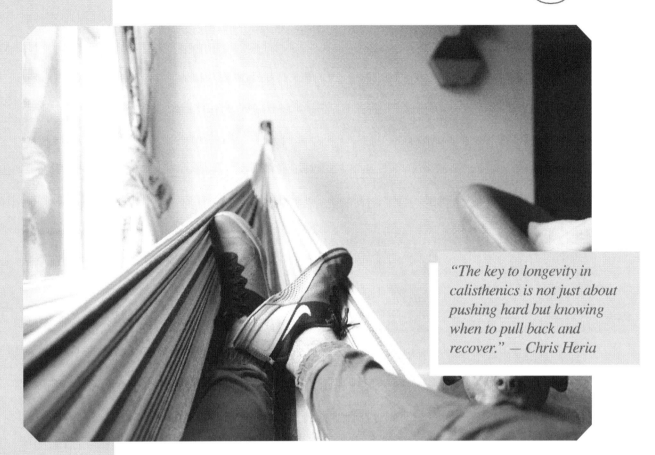

> *"The key to longevity in calisthenics is not just about pushing hard but knowing when to pull back and recover." — Chris Heria*

Imagine this: you've just finished an intense calisthenics workout, your muscles are pumped, and you feel that rush of accomplishment. But as you wipe the sweat from your brow, there's something crucial you might be overlooking—your recovery. You might think that training harder and longer will get you closer to your fitness goals, but what if I told you that recovery is the secret weapon that could make or break your progress?

Recovery isn't just about giving your body a break; it's about giving it the chance to rebuild, strengthen, and prepare for the next challenge. Whether you're a beginner or a seasoned calisthenics athlete, understanding the importance of recovery can significantly impact your performance, prevent injuries, and keep you on track for the long haul. So, let's dive into the world of recovery and injury prevention and uncover why these elements are essential to your calisthenics journey.

THE IMPORTANCE OF REST DAYS AND ACTIVE RECOVERY

WHEN YOU'RE PASSIONATE ABOUT YOUR CALISTHENICS ROUTINE, IT CAN BE TEMPTING TO PUSH YOURSELF EVERY DAY. HOWEVER, REST DAYS ARE NOT JUST OPTIONAL; THEY ARE AN INTEGRAL PART OF YOUR TRAINING PROGRAM. YOUR MUSCLES NEED TIME TO REPAIR AND GROW AFTER BEING STRESSED DURING EXERCISE. WHEN YOU WORK OUT, ESPECIALLY IN A DEMANDING DISCIPLINE LIKE CALISTHENICS, YOU CREATE TINY TEARS IN YOUR MUSCLE FIBERS.

These microtears are a normal part of the muscle-building process, but they need time to heal. Without adequate rest, your muscles don't get the chance to repair, which can lead to fatigue, decreased performance, and even injury.

Rest days aren't about being lazy; they're about being smart. Consider them as strategic pauses that allow your body to adapt to the physical demands you're placing on it. When you give your muscles time to recover, you enable them to grow stronger. This process is known as muscle hypertrophy, and it's the foundation of building strength and endurance in calisthenics.

ACTIVE RECOVERY: STAYING IN MOTION WITHOUT OVERDOING IT

Dr. Elizabeth Broad, a sports physiotherapist, emphasizes the importance of active recovery in preventing injuries. According to her, "Active recovery is a way to keep your body moving and your mind engaged while still allowing your muscles the time they need to repair. It's about striking the right balance between activity and rest."

While complete rest is essential, incorporating active recovery into your routine can also be incredibly beneficial. Active recovery involves low-intensity exercises that promote blood flow to your muscles without putting them under the same strain as your regular workouts. Activities like walking, swimming, yoga, or light cycling can help to flush out metabolic waste from your muscles, reduce soreness, and keep you moving without taxing your body.

Active recovery doesn't just help with physical recovery; it can also keep you mentally engaged in your fitness journey. It provides a way to maintain your routine and stay active while giving your body the care it needs. For instance, a gentle yoga session focused on stretching and breathing can be a great way to unwind both physically and mentally after a tough week of training.

STRETCHING AND MOBILITY FOR RECOVERY

STRETCHING IS OFTEN SEEN AS SOMETHING YOU DO BEFORE OR AFTER A WORKOUT TO WARM UP OR COOL DOWN. WHILE THAT'S CERTAINLY TRUE, STRETCHING PLAYS A MUCH LARGER ROLE IN RECOVERY AND INJURY PREVENTION. WHEN YOU STRETCH, YOU INCREASE THE FLEXIBILITY AND ELASTICITY OF YOUR MUSCLES AND CONNECTIVE TISSUES, WHICH CAN SIGNIFICANTLY REDUCE THE RISK OF INJURIES.

In calisthenics, where your body is the weight, flexibility, and mobility are crucial. Tight muscles can restrict your range of motion, leading to improper form and increasing the likelihood of injuries such as strains or sprains. Stretching helps to maintain and even improve your range of motion, ensuring that your joints and muscles can handle the demands of various exercises.

TYPES OF STRETCHING: STATIC VS. DYNAMIC

There are two main types of stretching: static and dynamic. Static stretching involves holding a stretch for an extended period, usually between 15 to 60 seconds. This type of stretching is best for post-workout routines as it helps to relax the muscles and improve flexibility. After a calisthenics session, static stretching can aid in lengthening the muscles that have been contracted during exercise, promoting a quicker recovery.

Dynamic stretching, on the other hand, involves moving parts of your body and gradually increasing reach, speed of movement, or both. This type of stretching is ideal for warming up before a workout because it prepares the muscles and joints for the activity ahead. In calisthenics, where fluid and controlled movements are key, dynamic stretching can enhance your performance by improving muscle coordination and reducing the risk of injury.

INCORPORATING MOBILITY WORK

Mobility work is another critical aspect of recovery, often overlooked in traditional training programs. Unlike flexibility, which refers to the length of a muscle, mobility is about the range of motion within your joints. Good mobility allows you to perform exercises with proper form, which is crucial in calisthenics, where technique is everything.

Mobility exercises can include joint rotations, resistance band work, and controlled articular rotations (CARs). These exercises help to lubricate the joints, improve circulation, and increase the range of motion. For example, shoulder mobility exercises can be particularly beneficial if you perform a lot of upper body calisthenics, like pull-ups or dips, as they help to prevent shoulder impingements and other injuries.

FOAM ROLLING AND SELF-MYOFASCIAL RELEASE TECHNIQUES

FOAM ROLLING HAS BECOME A POPULAR RECOVERY TOOL FOR ATHLETES AND FITNESS ENTHUSIASTS ALIKE, AND FOR A GOOD REASON. FOAM ROLLING IS A FORM OF SELF-MYOFASCIAL RELEASE (SMR), WHICH IS A TECHNIQUE USED TO RELEASE MUSCLE TIGHTNESS AND TRIGGER POINTS. WHEN YOU USE A FOAM ROLLER, YOU APPLY PRESSURE TO SPECIFIC AREAS OF YOUR BODY, HELPING TO BREAK UP ADHESIONS IN YOUR MUSCLES AND CONNECTIVE TISSUES. THESE ADHESIONS, OR "KNOTS," CAN RESTRICT MOVEMENT AND LEAD TO PAIN AND INJURY IF NOT ADDRESSED.

The benefits of foam rolling are extensive. It can improve blood circulation, increase flexibility, reduce muscle soreness, and enhance overall muscle performance. By regularly incorporating foam rolling into your recovery routine, you can maintain the health and function of your muscles, making your calisthenics practice more effective and enjoyable.

HOW TO USE A FOAM ROLLER EFFECTIVELY

It's important to use the correct technique to get the most out of foam rolling. Start by targeting major muscle groups like your back, quads, hamstrings, and calves. Slowly roll over the muscle, pausing on any tender spots for 20-30 seconds to allow the muscle to release.

Remember, foam rolling shouldn't be excruciatingly painful; if it is, you're likely applying too much pressure. The goal is to feel a deep tissue massage, not intense discomfort.

Incorporating foam rolling into your routine can be done either before or after your workouts. Pre-workout rolling can help to warm up the muscles and increase blood flow, making your workout more effective. Post-workout, it can aid in reducing muscle soreness and speeding up recovery by flushing out lactic acid and other metabolic waste products.

SELF-MYOFASCIAL RELEASE TECHNIQUES BEYOND FOAM ROLLING

While foam rolling is one of the most popular self-myofascial release techniques, there are other tools and methods you can use to achieve similar benefits. For example, massage balls, which are smaller and firmer than foam rollers, can be used to target smaller areas of the body, such as the shoulders, feet, or glutes. These tools allow you to apply more precise pressure to trigger points, helping to release tension and improve mobility.

Another technique is using a massage stick, which can be particularly useful for those who find foam rolling challenging. A massage stick allows for more controlled pressure and can be used to roll out muscle tension in areas that are harder to reach with a foam roller, like the calves or shins.

DEALING WITH COMMON INJURIES IN CALISTHENICS

DESPITE YOUR BEST EFFORTS TO PREVENT INJURIES, THEY CAN STILL HAPPEN, ESPECIALLY IN A DEMANDING DISCIPLINE LIKE CALISTHENICS. UNDERSTANDING HOW TO DEAL WITH COMMON INJURIES CAN HELP YOU RECOVER MORE QUICKLY AND GET BACK TO YOUR TRAINING WITH MINIMAL SETBACKS.

SHOULDER INJURIES: PREVENTION AND RECOVERY

Shoulder injuries are one of the most common issues faced by calisthenics athletes. The shoulder joint is incredibly versatile, but its range of motion also makes it vulnerable to injuries like impingements, rotator cuff tears, and tendinitis. These injuries often result from improper form, overuse, or insufficient warm-up.

Preventing shoulder injuries starts with proper warm-up routines and mobility work. Before engaging in upper body exercises, ensure that your shoulders are adequately warmed up with dynamic stretches and mobility drills. Additionally, focus on maintaining good posture and form during exercises like push-ups, pull-ups, and dips. Avoid letting your shoulders round forward, as this can place unnecessary strain on the joint.

If you do experience a shoulder injury, rest is crucial. Pushing through the pain can lead to more severe damage. Icing the affected area and performing gentle mobility exercises can help to reduce inflammation and maintain range of motion. As you recover, gradually reintroduce strength training exercises that target the rotator cuff muscles, as these are key to shoulder stability.

WRIST STRAINS: PREVENTION AND MANAGEMENT

Wrist strains are another common injury in calisthenics, especially for those who perform a lot of handstands, planches, or push-ups. The wrist joint is relatively small and not designed to bear heavy loads, making it susceptible to strains and sprains when not properly conditioned.

Preventing wrist injuries involves strengthening the muscles around the wrist and improving flexibility. Wrist stretches and strengthening exercises, such as wrist curls and extensions, should be a regular part of your training routine. Additionally, using wrist wraps or supports during high-load exercises can help to stabilize the joint and reduce the risk of injury.

If you experience a wrist strain, rest is essential. Avoid putting weight on the wrist until the pain subsides, and focus on mobility exercises to maintain flexibility. Gradually reintroduce weight-bearing exercises as your wrist heals, and consider modifying your technique or using supports to prevent future injuries.

LOWER BACK PAIN: PREVENTION AND RELIEF

Lower back pain is a common issue in calisthenics, often resulting from improper form, over-training, or a weak core. Exercises like squats, deadlifts, and leg raises can place significant strain on the lower back if not performed correctly.

To prevent lower back pain, focus on strengthening your core muscles, which provide stability and support for your spine. Incorporating exercises like planks, bird-dogs, and glute bridges into your routine can help to build a strong core and protect your lower back. Additionally, always prioritize proper form over the number of repetitions or the amount of weight you're lifting. Engage your core and keep your spine neutral to avoid placing unnecessary stress on your lower back.

If you do experience lower back pain, rest and gentle stretching are key. Avoid activities that exacerbate the pain and focus on exercises that promote spinal mobility, such as cat-cow stretches and pelvic tilts. As you recover, gradually reintroduce strength training exercises with an emphasis on proper form and core engagement.

HOW TO RECOVER FROM OVERTRAINING AND AVOID BURNOUT

OVERTRAINING OCCURS WHEN YOU PUSH YOUR BODY BEYOND ITS ABILITY TO RECOVER, LEADING TO A STATE OF CHRONIC FATIGUE, DECREASED PERFORMANCE, AND INCREASED RISK OF INJURY. THE SIGNS OF OVERTRAINING CAN BE SUBTLE AT FIRST BUT CAN ESCALATE IF NOT ADDRESSED. COMMON SYMPTOMS INCLUDE PERSISTENT MUSCLE SORENESS, FATIGUE, IRRITABILITY, INSOMNIA, AND A DECLINE IN WORKOUT PERFORMANCE.

It's important to listen to your body and recognize these signs early. Overtraining not only hampers your progress but can also lead to long-term health issues if not managed properly. If you notice that you're constantly tired, struggling to complete your workouts, or feeling unmotivated, it might be time to take a step back and reassess your training program.

STRATEGIES TO PREVENT BURNOUT

Preventing burnout starts with creating a balanced training program that includes sufficient rest and recovery. This means scheduling regular rest days, varying your workouts to avoid repetitive strain, and incorporating active recovery techniques like stretching, foam rolling, and light exercise.

Mental recovery is just as important as physical recovery. Taking time to relax, meditate, or engage in activities you enjoy outside of training can help to reduce stress and prevent burnout. Remember, your fitness journey should enhance your life, not dominate it. Maintaining a healthy balance between training, rest, and other aspects of your life is key to long-term success.

CREATING A RECOVERY PLAN

If you suspect that you might be overtraining, creating a structured recovery plan is essential. Start by reducing the intensity and frequency of your workouts to give your body a chance to heal. Focus on activities that promote relaxation and recovery, such as yoga, swimming, or gentle stretching.

Incorporate nutrition into your recovery plan by ensuring you're fueling your body with the right nutrients to support healing and energy production. Protein is particularly important for muscle repair, while carbohydrates help to replenish glycogen stores and provide energy. Hydration is also crucial, as dehydration can exacerbate symptoms of overtraining.

Finally, consider working with a coach or trainer to reassess your training program and ensure it's tailored to your individual needs and goals. A well-balanced program that prioritizes recovery will not only help you avoid burnout but will also enhance your overall performance and enjoyment of calisthenics.

THE BOTTOM LINE

Recovery and injury prevention are not just add-ons to your calisthenics routine—they are essential components of your fitness journey. By prioritizing rest, incorporating stretching and mobility work, using foam rolling techniques, and being mindful of common injuries, you can ensure that your body stays strong, resilient, and ready to take on new challenges.

Remember, progress in calisthenics isn't just about pushing harder or doing more; it's about training smarter. When you give your body the time and care it needs to recover, you're not just preventing injuries—you're setting yourself up for long-term success and sustainability in your fitness journey. So, embrace recovery as a vital part of your routine, and watch as your strength, flexibility, and overall performance soar to new heights.

THE MENTAL GAME OF CALISTHENICS

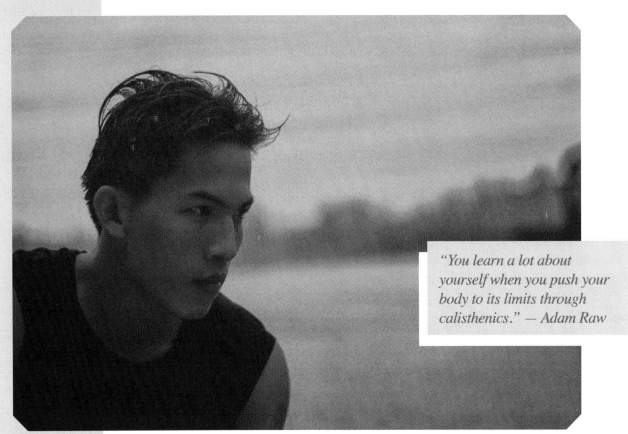

"You learn a lot about yourself when you push your body to its limits through calisthenics." — Adam Raw

Imagine yourself hanging from a pull-up bar, your muscles burning as you strive to complete just one more rep. The physical challenge is undeniable, but what often goes unnoticed is the mental struggle that accompanies it. Calisthenics is as much a mental game as it is a physical one. In fact, your mindset can be the determining factor between giving up and pushing through to new levels of strength and endurance. Understanding and mastering the mental aspects of calisthenics can transform your approach to training, making it not just a way to build your body but a powerful tool for developing resilience, focus, and discipline in every area of your life.

This chapter will guide you through the mental challenges unique to calisthenics and provide you with strategies to overcome them. Whether you're just starting out or you're an experienced practitioner looking to advance to the next level, these mental techniques will help you break through barriers, stay motivated, and achieve your long-term goals. Let's explore how building mental toughness, visualizing success, practicing mindfulness, and developing consistency can elevate your calisthenics practice and your overall well-being.

BUILDING MENTAL TOUGHNESS: OVERCOMING BARRIERS AND STAYING MOTIVATED

THE FIRST STEP IN MASTERING THE MENTAL GAME OF CALISTHENICS IS BUILDING MENTAL TOUGH-NESS. THIS ISN'T JUST ABOUT GRITTING YOUR TEETH AND PUSHING THROUGH THE PAIN—THOUGH THAT'S PART OF IT. MENTAL TOUGHNESS IS ABOUT DEVELOPING THE RESILIENCE TO OVERCOME OBSTACLES, WHETHER THEY'RE PHYSICAL, EMOTIONAL, OR PSYCHOLOGICAL. IT'S ABOUT STAYING MOTIVATED EVEN WHEN PROGRESS SEEMS SLOW AND FINDING THE STRENGTH TO KEEP GOING WHEN YOUR BODY IS TELLING YOU TO QUIT.

UNDERSTANDING MENTAL TOUGHNESS

Mental toughness is often misunderstood as simply being about willpower. But it's much more than that. It's about how you handle setbacks, how you respond to failure, and how you manage the inevitable plateaus that come with any long-term training program. In calisthenics, where progress can sometimes be frustratingly slow, mental toughness is what keeps you going.

A study conducted by Clough et al. (2002) on mental toughness outlines four key components: control, commitment, challenge, and confidence. These components are essential in calisthenics. Control refers to your ability to remain calm and focused, even under pressure. Commitment is your ability to set goals and stick to them, no matter what. Challenge is about seeing obstacles as opportunities to grow rather than insurmountable barriers. Finally, confidence is about believing in your ability to overcome challenges and achieve your goals.

OVERCOMING BARRIERS

One of the biggest barriers in calisthenics is self-doubt. You might find yourself thinking, "I'll never be able to do a muscle-up," or "I'm just not strong enough." These thoughts are normal, but they can be incredibly limiting. The key to overcoming them is to shift your mindset from one of limitation to one of possibility.

Instead of focusing on what you can't do, focus on what you can do. Break down your goals into smaller, manageable steps. If a muscle-up seems impossible, start by mastering the pull-up. Once you've built up your strength, work on your explosive power. Each small victory will build your confidence and bring you closer to your ultimate goal.

STAYING MOTIVATED

Staying motivated in calisthenics can be challenging, especially when progress feels slow. But motivation isn't something that just happens—it's something you have to cultivate. One of the best ways to stay motivated is to connect with your "why." Why did you start calisthenics in the first place? What are you hoping to achieve? Whether it's improving your physical fitness, mastering a new skill, or simply challenging yourself, keeping your "why" at the forefront of your mind can help you stay motivated, even when the going gets tough.

Another powerful tool for staying motivated is to celebrate your progress, no matter how small. Every time you hit a new personal best, whether it's one more pull-up or holding a plank for a few extra seconds, take a moment to acknowledge your progress. These small wins can add up to big changes over time.

THE NEW CALISTHENICS FORMULA

VISUALIZATION TECHNIQUES FOR SUCCESS IN ADVANCED MOVEMENTS

ONCE YOU'VE BUILT MENTAL TOUGHNESS, THE NEXT STEP IS TO HARNESS THE POWER OF VISUALIZATION. VISUALIZATION IS A POWERFUL TOOL USED BY ELITE ATHLETES IN EVERY SPORT TO ENHANCE PERFORMANCE, AND IT'S JUST AS EFFECTIVE IN CALISTHENICS.

WHAT IS VISUALIZATION?

Visualization, also known as mental imagery, is the process of creating a mental image of a specific event or outcome. When you visualize yourself performing a movement, your brain activates the same neural pathways as it would if you were actually performing the movement. This means that visualization can help you improve your skills, build confidence, and prepare your mind for the challenges ahead.

A famous example of visualization in sports comes from Olympic swimmer Michael Phelps, who used visualization techniques to mentally rehearse his races down to the smallest detail. He would visualize everything from his starting dive to his final stroke, preparing his mind for every possible scenario. This mental preparation was a key factor in his success.

APPLYING VISUALIZATION TO CALISTHENICS

In calisthenics, visualization can be particularly useful for mastering advanced movements like the muscle-up, handstand, or front lever. These movements require not only physical strength but also a high level of coordination and body awareness. Visualization can help you mentally rehearse these movements, making them feel more familiar and achievable.

To use visualization in your practice, start by finding a quiet place where you won't be disturbed. Close your eyes and take a few deep breaths to calm your mind. Then, visualize yourself performing the movement you're working on. Imagine every detail—the position of your body, the engagement of your muscles, the feeling of control as you execute the movement. Try to make the image as vivid and realistic as possible.

You can also use visualization to prepare for your workouts. Before you start your training session, take a few minutes to visualize yourself completing the workout. Picture yourself performing each exercise with perfect form, feeling strong and focused throughout. This mental preparation can help you enter your workout with a positive mindset and a clear sense of purpose.

THE ROLE OF MINDFULNESS AND FOCUS IN BODYWEIGHT TRAINING

MINDFULNESS AND FOCUS ARE ESSENTIAL COMPONENTS OF THE MENTAL GAME OF CALISTHENICS. WHEN YOU'RE FULLY PRESENT IN THE MOMENT, YOU'RE ABLE TO PERFORM AT YOUR BEST, BOTH PHYSICALLY AND MENTALLY.

WHAT IS MINDFULNESS?

Mindfulness is the practice of paying attention to the present moment without judgment. It's about being fully aware of your thoughts, feelings, and sensations as they arise without getting caught up in them. In the context of calisthenics, mindfulness means being fully present during your workouts, paying attention to your body, your breath, and your movements.

Mindfulness has been shown to have numerous benefits for athletes, including improved focus, reduced stress, and better performance. A study by Kabat-Zinn et al. (1992) found that mindfulness-based stress reduction (MBSR) can lead to significant improvements in athletic performance, as well as overall well-being.

APPLYING MINDFULNESS TO CALISTHENICS

In calisthenics, mindfulness can help you stay focused and avoid distractions. When you're mindful, you're less likely to be thrown off by negative thoughts or external distractions. Instead, you can maintain a steady focus on your movements, ensuring that each rep is performed with intention and control.

To practice mindfulness during your workouts, start by focusing on your breath. Take a few deep breaths before you begin your workout, and continue to focus on your breath throughout your training session. If your mind starts to wander, gently bring your attention back to your breath and your movements.

Another way to practice mindfulness is to perform each exercise with full awareness. Instead of rushing through your reps, take your time to feel each movement. Notice how your muscles engage, how your body moves through space, and how your breath supports your movements. This level of awareness can help you perform each exercise with better form and greater control.

ENHANCING FOCUS

Focus is closely related to mindfulness, but it's more about directing your attention to a specific task or goal. In calisthenics, focus is crucial for mastering complex movements and achieving your goals.

One technique for enhancing focus is to set a clear intention for each workout. Before you begin your training session, decide what you want to achieve. It could be mastering a specific movement, improving your form, or simply getting through the workout with maximum effort. By setting a clear intention, you can direct your focus toward that goal, making it easier to stay on track.

Another way to enhance focus is to eliminate distractions. This might mean putting your phone on silent, finding a quiet place to work out, or using noise-canceling headphones to block out background noise. The fewer distractions you have, the easier it will be to maintain your focus.

DEVELOPING DISCIPLINE AND CONSISTENCY IN YOUR PRACTICE

DISCIPLINE AND CONSISTENCY ARE THE CORNERSTONES OF SUCCESS IN CALISTHENICS. NO MATTER HOW MOTIVATED YOU ARE, IF YOU DON'T HAVE THE DISCIPLINE TO STICK TO YOUR TRAINING PLAN AND THE CONSISTENCY TO KEEP SHOWING UP, YOU'LL STRUGGLE TO MAKE PROGRESS.

THE IMPORTANCE OF DISCIPLINE

Discipline is about doing what needs to be done, even when you don't feel like it. It's about sticking to your training plan, even when you're tired, busy, or just not in the mood. In calisthenics, where progress can be slow and the workouts can be challenging, discipline is essential.

One way to build discipline is to create a routine. When you have a set routine, it becomes easier to stay consistent because you don't have to rely on motivation alone. For example, if you always train at the same time each day, it becomes a habit, and you're less likely to skip your workout.

Another way to build discipline is to set clear, achievable goals. When you have a specific goal in mind, it's easier to stay focused and committed. For example, if your goal is to achieve your first muscle-up, you'll be more motivated to stick to your training plan because you know that each workout brings you closer to that goal.

THE POWER OF CONSISTENCY

Consistency is just as important as discipline. Even the best training plan won't work if you're not consistent. In calisthenics, consistency is key to building strength, improving your skills, and making progress.

One of the biggest challenges to consistency is staying motivated over the long term. It's easy to stay motivated when you're seeing progress, but what happens when you hit a plateau? This is where discipline comes in. Even when progress is slow, if you're consistent, you'll eventually break through that plateau and start seeing results again.

A great way to stay consistent is to track your progress. Keep a training journal where you record your workouts, your progress, and your thoughts and feelings about your training. This can help you stay accountable and motivated because you can see how far you've come and how much progress you've made.

HOW TO SET AND ACHIEVE LONG-TERM CALISTHENICS GOALS

SETTING AND ACHIEVING LONG-TERM GOALS IS A CRUCIAL PART OF THE MENTAL GAME OF CALISTHENICS. WITHOUT CLEAR GOALS, IT'S EASY TO LOSE FOCUS AND MOTIVATION. BUT WITH THE RIGHT GOALS IN PLACE, YOU CAN STAY ON TRACK AND MAKE CONSISTENT PROGRESS.

SETTING SMART GOALS

When it comes to goal setting, one of the most effective techniques is to use the SMART framework. SMART stands for Specific, Measurable, Achievable, Relevant, and Time-bound. Let's break down each of these components:

- **Specific:** Your goals should be clear and specific so you know exactly what you're working towards. Instead of saying, "I want to get stronger," set a specific goal like, "I want to be able to do ten consecutive pull-ups."

- **Measurable:** Your goals should be measurable so you can track your progress and know when you've achieved them. In the pull-up example, you can measure your progress by counting how many pull-ups you can do each week.

- **Achievable:** Your goals should be challenging but achievable. If you're just starting out, aiming for ten pull-ups might be too ambitious, so start with a smaller goal and work your way up.

- **Relevant:** Your goals should be relevant to your overall objectives. If your main focus is building upper body strength, then a pull-up goal is relevant. But if your focus is on improving flexibility, you might want to set a different goal.

- **Time-bound:** Your goals should have a deadline so you have a sense of urgency and can create a timeline for your progress. For example, you might set a goal to achieve ten pull-ups within three months.

BREAKING DOWN LONG-TERM GOALS

Long-term goals can sometimes feel overwhelming, especially if they require a lot of time and effort. One way to make them more manageable is to break them down into smaller, short-term goals. For example, if your long-term goal is to achieve a front lever, you could break it down into smaller goals like improving your core strength, mastering the tuck front lever, and gradually progressing to the full front lever.

By breaking down your long-term goals into smaller steps, you can focus on making consistent progress rather than getting overwhelmed by the size of the goal. Each time you achieve a short-term goal, you'll feel a sense of accomplishment, which can help keep you motivated and on track.

STAYING COMMITTED TO YOUR GOALS

Setting goals is the easy part—staying committed to them is where the real challenge lies. One of the biggest obstacles to goal achievement is losing focus or motivation over time. To stay committed to your goals, it's important to regularly revisit them and remind yourself of why you set them in the first place.

Another key to staying committed is to stay flexible. Life is unpredictable, and sometimes things don't go according to plan. If you encounter obstacles or setbacks, it's important to adjust your goals and your approach, rather than giving up. For example, if you experience an injury, you might need to adjust your training plan and set new goals that accommodate your recovery.

Finally, it's important to celebrate your successes along the way. Each time you achieve a goal, take a moment to acknowledge your hard work and celebrate your progress. This can help keep you motivated and focused on the bigger picture.

THE BOTTOM LINE

The mental game of calisthenics is just as important as the physical game. By building mental toughness, using visualization techniques, practicing mindfulness, developing discipline and consistency, and setting and achieving long-term goals, you can unlock your full potential in calisthenics. However, perhaps the most important aspect of the mental game is cultivating a strong mind-body connection. When your mind and body are working together in harmony, you'll not only achieve your goals, but you'll also experience the deeper benefits of calisthenics, such as improved focus, reduced stress, and a greater sense of well-being.

So, the next time you step up to the bar or get down on the floor for a set of push-ups, remember that calisthenics is not just a physical practice—it's a mental one, too. By mastering the mental game, you'll not only become stronger and more skilled, but you'll also develop the resilience, focus, and confidence to overcome any challenge that comes your way.

CALISTHENICS AND FUNCTIONAL STRENGTH FOR EVERYDAY LIFE

11

CHAPTER

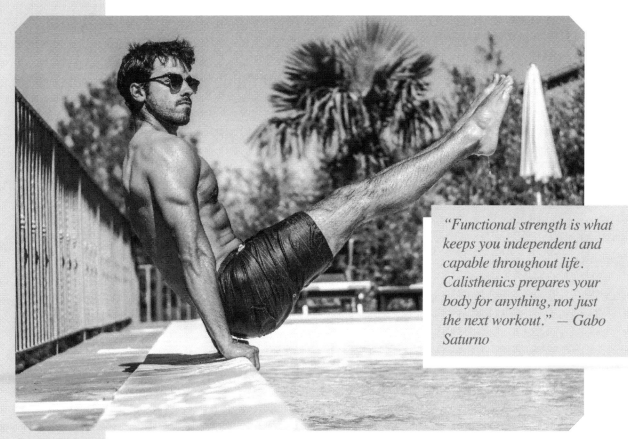

> *"Functional strength is what keeps you independent and capable throughout life. Calisthenics prepares your body for anything, not just the next workout."* — *Gabo Saturno*

Imagine moving through your day with effortless strength and grace, whether you're picking up a heavy box, playing with your kids, or simply getting out of bed in the morning. This isn't some distant fantasy—it's the reality you can achieve by incorporating calisthenics into your life. Calisthenics isn't just about building muscle or looking good, though those are nice bonuses. It's about developing the kind of strength that truly matters—the kind that makes your everyday life easier, more efficient, and, ultimately, more enjoyable.

In this chapter, we'll dive into how calisthenics goes beyond aesthetics to enhance your functional strength, mobility, and overall well-being. We'll explore why this form of exercise is uniquely suited to prepare your body for the demands of daily life, and how you can integrate it seamlessly into your routine. Whether you're a seasoned athlete or someone just beginning your fitness journey, the insights here will help you build a body that doesn't just look strong but is strong in all the ways that count.

THE REAL-LIFE APPLICATIONS OF CALISTHENICS STRENGTH

WHEN YOU THINK ABOUT STRENGTH TRAINING, YOU MIGHT PICTURE HEAVY WEIGHTS, MACHINES, OR PERHAPS ENDLESS REPS IN THE GYM. BUT THE TRUTH IS, STRENGTH ISN'T JUST ABOUT HOW MUCH YOU CAN BENCH PRESS OR DEADLIFT—IT'S ABOUT HOW WELL YOUR BODY CAN PERFORM THE TASKS YOU NEED IT TO, DAY IN AND DAY OUT. THIS IS WHERE CALISTHENICS SHINES. BY USING YOUR BODY WEIGHT AS RESISTANCE, CALISTHENICS BUILDS A KIND OF STRENGTH THAT'S HIGHLY FUNCTIONAL— STRENGTH THAT DIRECTLY TRANSLATES TO BETTER PERFORMANCE IN YOUR DAILY ACTIVITIES.

EVERYDAY STRENGTH THAT MATTERS

Consider the simple act of lifting a bag of groceries, climbing stairs, or even getting up from the floor. These are movements we all do regularly, yet they require a combination of strength, balance, and coordination that traditional weightlifting doesn't always address. Calisthenics, however, targets these exact qualities. Exercises like push-ups, squats, and planks mimic the natural movements of your body, training not just your muscles but also your tendons, ligaments, and joints to work together more efficiently.

For instance, a push-up isn't just an upper-body workout; it's a full-body exercise that engages your core, stabilizes your shoulder joints, and improves your posture—all essential elements when you're carrying heavy items or performing tasks that require upper-body strength. Similarly, a squat strengthens your legs and core while improving your balance, making activities like bending down to pick something up or standing from a seated position much easier.

BUILDING RESILIENCE FOR LIFE'S CHALLENGES

Beyond these everyday tasks, calisthenics helps build resilience against the physical challenges life throws your way. Think about how often you twist, turn, or reach for something in your daily routine. Each of these movements engages multiple muscle groups and requires a level of coordination that isolated weightlifting exercises might not develop. Calisthenics exercises, on the other hand, are compound movements that train your body to move as a cohesive unit, improving your overall movement efficiency and reducing the risk of injury.

For example, the burpee—a classic calisthenics exercise—combines a squat, push-up, and jump into one fluid movement. This not only improves your cardiovascular fitness but also enhances your agility, coordination, and full-body strength. The more adept you become at such exercises, the better equipped you are to handle the physical demands of daily life, from chasing after your kids to tackling that unexpected home improvement project.

CALISTHENICS: A LIFELONG INVESTMENT IN HEALTH

The beauty of calisthenics lies in its simplicity and accessibility. You don't need a gym membership, expensive equipment, or even a lot of space to get started. All you need is your body and the willingness to move it in ways that challenge and strengthen it. This makes calisthenics a sustainable form of exercise that you can practice well into your later years, helping you maintain your independence and quality of life for as long as possible.

FUNCTIONAL MOVEMENT PATTERNS AND THEIR BENEFITS BEYOND FITNESS

WE OFTEN TAKE FOR GRANTED THE ABILITY TO MOVE FREELY, BUT AS WE AGE OR IF WE BECOME INJURED, WE QUICKLY REALIZE JUST HOW CRUCIAL FUNCTIONAL MOVEMENT IS. FUNCTIONAL MOVEMENT REFERS TO THE ABILITY TO PERFORM NATURAL, EVERYDAY ACTIONS LIKE BENDING, TWISTING, LIFTING, AND REACHING WITHOUT PAIN OR DIFFICULTY. CALISTHENICS IS PARTICULARLY EFFECTIVE AT IMPROVING THESE MOVEMENT PATTERNS, MAKING IT AN INVALUABLE TOOL FOR ANYONE LOOKING TO MAINTAIN OR ENHANCE THEIR FUNCTIONAL FITNESS.

UNDERSTANDING FUNCTIONAL MOVEMENT

At its core, functional movement is about training your body to work as a whole rather than in isolated parts. In contrast to traditional strength training, which often focuses on individual muscle groups, functional movement exercises are designed to engage multiple muscle groups simultaneously. This not only builds strength but also improves balance, coordination, and flexibility—all of which are essential for performing daily tasks with ease.

Take, for example, the exercise known as the "lunge." While it primarily targets your legs, it also engages your core, improves your balance, and mimics the natural movement of stepping forward or backward—actions you perform countless times each day. By regularly practicing lunges, you're training your body to move more efficiently, which can reduce the risk of injury and make everyday activities like walking, running, or even standing more comfortable.

ENHANCING BALANCE AND COORDINATION

Balance and coordination are often overlooked aspects of fitness, yet they are crucial for maintaining independence and preventing injuries, especially as we age. Calisthenics exercises are particularly effective at improving these areas because they require you to stabilize your body while performing movements.

For instance, exercises like single-leg squats or the "pistol squat" challenge your balance and force you to engage your stabilizer muscles—those small but mighty muscles that support your joints and help you maintain your balance. By strengthening these muscles, you improve your overall stability, which can help prevent falls and other common injuries.

FLEXIBILITY: THE UNSUNG HERO OF FUNCTIONAL MOVEMENT

Flexibility plays a vital role in functional movement by allowing your joints to move through their full range of motion without restriction. Calisthenics naturally improves flexibility because many exercises involve dynamic stretching, which helps lengthen and strengthen your muscles simultaneously.

A great example of this is the "inchworm" exercise, where you start in a standing position, bend forward to touch the floor, walk your hands out into a plank position, and then walk your feet forward to meet your hands. This movement stretches your hamstrings, calves, and lower back while also strengthening your core and shoulders. By incorporating such exercises into your routine, you not only improve your flexibility but also ensure that your muscles and joints remain limber and functional.

LONG-TERM BENEFITS OF FUNCTIONAL MOVEMENT TRAINING

The benefits of improving your functional movement patterns extend far beyond fitness. When your body moves more efficiently, you're less likely to experience pain or discomfort during everyday activities, and you're better equipped to handle the physical demands of life as you age. Whether it's reaching for something on a high shelf, bending down to tie your shoes, or carrying groceries from the car, functional movement training helps you perform these tasks with ease and confidence.

Moreover, by focusing on functional movement, you're investing in your long-term health and well-being. As your balance, coordination, and flexibility improve, so does your overall quality of life. You'll find that you have more energy, fewer aches and pains, and a greater sense of physical freedom—all of which contribute to a happier, healthier you.

TRAINING FOR MOBILITY, FLEXIBILITY, AND LONGEVITY

IN THE WORLD OF FITNESS, THERE'S OFTEN A HEAVY EMPHASIS ON BUILDING MUSCLE AND BURNING FAT. WHILE THESE GOALS ARE IMPORTANT, THEY SHOULDN'T COME AT THE EXPENSE OF MOBILITY AND FLEXIBILITY—TWO KEY COMPONENTS OF LONGEVITY AND OVERALL HEALTH. MOBILITY REFERS TO THE ABILITY OF YOUR JOINTS TO MOVE FREELY THROUGH THEIR FULL RANGE OF MOTION, WHILE FLEXIBILITY IS THE LENGTH AND ELASTICITY OF THE MUSCLES THAT SUPPORT THOSE JOINTS. TOGETHER, THESE ELEMENTS ARE ESSENTIAL FOR MAINTAINING A HEALTHY, FUNCTIONAL BODY THROUGHOUT YOUR LIFE.

THE ROLE OF MOBILITY IN EVERYDAY LIFE

Mobility is crucial for performing even the simplest of tasks, such as reaching for something on a high shelf, bending down to pick up an object, or turning your head to look over your shoulder. Without sufficient mobility, these movements can become difficult, painful, or even impossible, leading to a decrease in your quality of life.

Calisthenics exercises are particularly effective at improving mobility because they involve dynamic movements that require your joints to move through their full range of motion. For example, exercises like "hip circles" or "arm swings" help to lubricate your joints, increase blood flow, and improve the flexibility of the surrounding muscles, all of which contribute to better mobility.

FLEXIBILITY: THE FOUNDATION OF PAIN-FREE MOVEMENT

Flexibility is often seen as the domain of yogis and dancers, but it's actually a crucial component of any well-rounded fitness routine. Without adequate flexibility, your muscles can become tight and short, leading to imbalances that can cause pain, limit your range of motion, and increase your risk of injury.

Incorporating flexibility training into your calisthenics routine can help prevent these issues and improve your overall movement quality. Simple exercises like "toe touches" or "quad stretches" can go a long way in lengthening your muscles and reducing tension, making everyday movements smoother and more comfortable.

LONGEVITY THROUGH MOVEMENT

One of the most significant benefits of focusing on mobility and flexibility is the impact it has on your longevity. As we age, our joints naturally lose some of their mobility, and our muscles tend to become stiffer and less pliable. This can lead to a decrease in functional movement, making everyday tasks more challenging and increasing the risk of falls and other injuries.

However, by regularly practicing calisthenics, you can slow down or even reverse these effects. Studies have shown that maintaining mobility and flexibility as you age can help you stay active, independent, and pain-free well into your later years. This means you can continue doing the things you love—whether it's playing with your grandchildren, traveling, or simply enjoying a walk in the park—without being held back by your body.

INTEGRATING MOBILITY AND FLEXIBILITY INTO YOUR ROUTINE

The best way to ensure you're getting enough mobility and flexibility training is to incorporate it into your daily routine. This doesn't mean you need to spend hours stretching or doing mobility drills; even just a few minutes a day can make a significant difference.

Start your day with a simple stretching routine that targets your major muscle groups, such as your hamstrings, quadriceps, and shoulders. You can also include mobility exercises like "leg swings" or "spinal twists" to get your joints moving and increase your range of motion. Don't forget to warm up before your workouts and cool down afterward with some gentle stretching to keep your muscles and joints healthy and flexible.

HOW TO INCORPORATE CALISTHENICS INTO OTHER SPORTS AND ACTIVITIES

WHILE CALISTHENICS IS AN EXCELLENT STANDALONE FORM OF EXERCISE, IT'S ALSO INCREDIBLY VERSATILE AND CAN BE EASILY INTEGRATED INTO OTHER SPORTS AND ACTIVITIES. WHETHER YOU'RE A RUNNER, A SWIMMER, OR A MARTIAL ARTIST, CALISTHENICS CAN HELP YOU IMPROVE YOUR PERFORMANCE, REDUCE YOUR RISK OF INJURY, AND ENHANCE YOUR OVERALL ATHLETICISM.

ENHANCING ATHLETIC PERFORMANCE

One of the primary benefits of incorporating calisthenics into your training routine is the improvement in your overall athletic performance. Calisthenics exercises are functional by nature, meaning they train your body to move more efficiently and effectively. This translates to better performance in virtually any sport or physical activity.

For example, if you're a runner, calisthenics can help you build strength in your legs, core, and upper body, which are all essential for maintaining proper form and reducing fatigue during long runs. Exercises like "mountain climbers" and "plank variations" target your core and improve your stability, helping you maintain good posture and avoid injury.

If you're a swimmer, calisthenics can help you develop the upper body and core strength needed to power through the water with speed and efficiency. Exercises like "push-ups" and "pull-ups" strengthen your shoulders, chest, and back, giving you the power and endurance to swim longer and faster.

REDUCING THE RISK OF INJURY

Injuries are a common concern for athletes, and they can often be caused by imbalances, weaknesses, or a lack of flexibility. Calisthenics can help address these issues by providing a balanced workout that targets all the major muscle groups and improves your overall movement quality.

For instance, if you're a soccer player, you might be prone to ankle or knee injuries due to the high-impact nature of the sport. Incorporating calisthenics exercises like "single-leg squats" or "calf raises" into your routine can help strengthen the muscles around your joints, improving your stability and reducing your risk of injury.

Similarly, if you're a martial artist, you need a high level of flexibility, agility, and strength to perform at your best. Calisthenics exercises like "burpees" or "jump squats" can help you develop explosive power, while exercises like "hip openers" or "spinal twists" can improve your flexibility and prevent injuries.

SUPPORTING A WELL-ROUNDED, ACTIVE LIFESTYLE

Beyond the physical benefits, integrating calisthenics into your other activities can help you develop a more well-rounded, active lifestyle. Calisthenics provides a unique combination of strength, flexibility, and endurance training, making it the perfect complement to virtually any sport or physical activity.

For example, if you enjoy hiking, calisthenics can help you build the lower body and core strength needed to tackle steep inclines and rough terrain. Exercises like "step-ups" or "glute bridges" can strengthen your legs and hips, improving your stamina and reducing your risk of injury on the trail.

If you're into yoga, calisthenics can help you build the strength and stability needed to hold challenging poses and improve your overall practice. Exercises like "planks" or "side planks" target your core and improve your balance, helping you maintain proper alignment and prevent injuries.

CREATING A BALANCED TRAINING ROUTINE

It's important to create a balanced routine that incorporates both your sport-specific activities and calisthenics exercises to get the most out of your training. This will help you develop the strength, flexibility, and endurance needed to excel in your chosen activity while also reducing your risk of injury and improving your overall athleticism.

Start by identifying the key muscle groups and movement patterns that are important for your sport or activity. Then, select calisthenics exercises that target those areas and incorporate them into your training routine. For example, if you're a cyclist, focus on exercises that strengthen your legs, core, and lower back, such as "squats," "planks," and "back extensions."

Remember to also include mobility and flexibility exercises in your routine to ensure that your muscles and joints remain healthy and functional. This will help you move more efficiently, reduce your risk of injury, and enhance your overall performance.

THE POWER OF CONSISTENCY

Like any form of exercise, the key to success with calisthenics is consistency. To see real results, you need to make calisthenics a regular part of your training routine. This doesn't mean you have to spend hours each day doing push-ups and squats—just a few minutes of focused, intentional movement each day can make a significant difference in your overall strength, flexibility, and athletic performance.

By incorporating calisthenics into your daily routine, you'll not only improve your physical fitness but also develop a greater sense of body awareness and control. This will help you move through your day with greater ease, confidence, and resilience, allowing you to enjoy all the activities you love with less pain and more joy.

THE BOTTOM LINE

Calisthenics offers you more than just a path to physical fitness—it gives you the tools to build a body that is strong, flexible, and capable of handling the demands of everyday life. By focusing on functional movement patterns, mobility, and flexibility, calisthenics prepares you for the real-life challenges that come your way, whether it's lifting heavy objects, maintaining your balance on uneven terrain, or simply moving through your day with greater ease and comfort.

As you integrate calisthenics into your fitness routine, you'll begin to notice improvements not just in your physical appearance but in how you feel and move throughout your daily life. You'll develop the kind of strength that truly matters—the kind that enhances your quality of life and allows you to live more fully and actively, no matter what your age or fitness level.

So start today and embrace the power of calisthenics. Your future self will thank you for it.

STAYING CONSISTENT AND ADAPTING TO YOUR LIFESTYLE

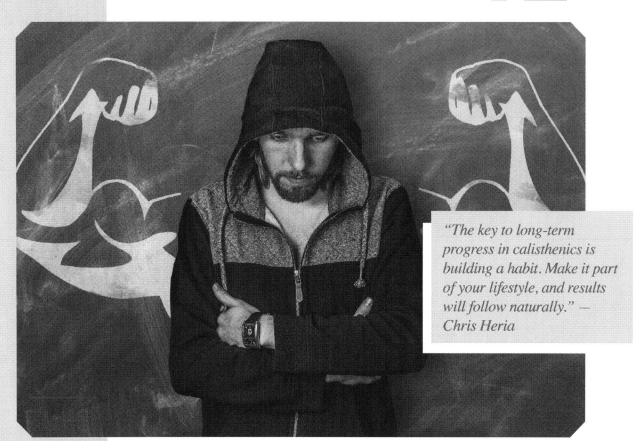

"The key to long-term progress in calisthenics is building a habit. Make it part of your lifestyle, and results will follow naturally." — Chris Heria

When it comes to fitness, consistency is key. You've likely heard this before, but what does it really mean to be consistent, especially when life gets in the way?

Between work, family, and the endless to-do lists that seem to multiply overnight, finding time for regular exercise can feel like an impossible task. Yet, staying active is one of the most important things you can do for your long-term health and well-being.

This chapter is your guide to integrating calisthenics into your daily life, no matter how busy you are. It's about creating a routine that works for you, keeping your motivation high, and adapting when necessary. Let's dive into how you can make fitness a sustainable part of your lifestyle.

CREATING A WORKOUT SCHEDULE THAT FITS YOUR LIFE

WHEN YOU FIRST DIVE INTO CALISTHENICS, ITS SHEER FLEXIBILITY—NO PUN INTENDED—CAN BE BOTH A BLESSING AND A CURSE. THE FREEDOM TO WORK OUT ANYWHERE, WITHOUT THE NEED FOR EQUIPMENT, IS LIBERATING. HOWEVER, WITHOUT A STRUCTURED PLAN, IT'S EASY TO LET DAYS SLIP BY WITHOUT DOING ANYTHING AT ALL. SO, HOW DO YOU CREATE A WORKOUT SCHEDULE THAT NOT ONLY FITS INTO YOUR LIFE BUT ALSO BECOMES A NON-NEGOTIABLE PART OF IT?

FINDING YOUR OPTIMAL TIME

The first step in creating a workout schedule that sticks is to find the time of day that works best for you. Are you a morning person who feels energized by the crisp air and the promise of a new day? Or do you find your energy peaks in the evening, when you can unwind after a day's work? Understanding your natural rhythms will help you identify when you're most likely to stick with your workouts.

Studies suggest that people who exercise in the morning are more consistent in their routines, as it's easier to knock out a workout before the demands of the day start piling up. However, if mornings are a struggle, there's no need to force it. What matters most is consistency, so choose a time when you're likely to be both mentally and physically ready to exercise. If your schedule varies, don't be afraid to adjust your workout times. Flexibility is key to maintaining long-term adherence.

DESIGNING A BALANCED ROUTINE

Once you've identified your optimal workout time, the next step is to design a balanced routine that you can stick to. A well-rounded calisthenics routine typically includes a mix of strength training, flexibility exercises, and cardiovascular activities. The beauty of calisthenics is that many exercises can target multiple areas at once. For example, a routine that includes push-ups, squats, and planks covers your upper body, lower body, and core in one go.

To make your routine more sustainable, consider starting with shorter, more frequent sessions. For instance, instead of committing to an hour-long workout three times a week, try 20-minute sessions five days a week. This approach not only makes it easier to fit workouts into your day but also helps build a habit. As the saying goes, "The best workout is the one you actually do."

Dr. James Levine, a professor of medicine at the Mayo Clinic, suggests breaking up your workouts into smaller segments if you're pressed for time. He says, "It's not about having a full hour to work out; it's about making use of the time you do have. Even a few minutes of exercise here and there can add up."

FLEXIBILITY IS KEY

Life is unpredictable, and there will be days when your planned workout doesn't happen. That's okay. The key is to be flexible and not let one missed workout derail your entire routine. If you can't fit in a full session, do a quick 10-minute workout or some stretching to keep the habit going. The goal is to stay consistent over time, not to be perfect every day.

THE NEW CALISTHENICS FORMULA

INCORPORATING REST AND RECOVERY

One mistake many people make when creating a workout schedule is overlooking the importance of rest. In calisthenics, as with any form of exercise, your body needs time to recover. Without adequate rest, you risk injury and burnout, both of which can derail your progress. Aim to include at least one or two rest days in your weekly schedule. On these days, you can engage in light activities such as walking or stretching, which promote recovery without putting undue stress on your muscles.

HOW TO STAY MOTIVATED LONG-TERM

STARTING A NEW WORKOUT ROUTINE IS OFTEN THE EASIEST PART. THE INITIAL EXCITEMENT FUELS YOUR MOTIVATION, AND YOU CAN'T WAIT TO SEE RESULTS. BUT AS TIME GOES ON, THAT EXCITEMENT CAN WANE, AND STICKING TO YOUR ROUTINE BECOMES MORE OF A CHALLENGE. STAYING MOTIVATED LONG-TERM REQUIRES MORE THAN JUST WILLPOWER; IT REQUIRES STRATEGIES TO KEEP YOUR GOALS FRESH AND YOUR WORKOUTS ENJOYABLE.

FIND YOUR "WHY"

Understanding your motivation for working out is crucial. Why did you start this journey? Was it to improve your health, gain confidence, or simply feel better in your own skin? Whatever your reason, keep it front and center. Write it down, put it somewhere visible, and remind yourself of it regularly. This will help you stay focused when the going gets tough.

SET MEANINGFUL GOALS

One of the most powerful tools for maintaining long-term motivation is goal-setting. But it's not just about setting any goals; it's about setting meaningful goals that resonate with you personally. Instead of focusing solely on aesthetic goals like losing weight or building muscle, consider setting functional goals, such as mastering a new calisthenics move, increasing your endurance, or improving your flexibility.

Research shows that goals related to personal growth and self-improvement are more likely to sustain long-term motivation than those tied to external rewards or pressures. For example, aiming to do ten pull-ups in a row or holding a handstand for 30 seconds can be incredibly motivating because they represent tangible progress. Each small victory along the way reinforces your commitment and keeps you engaged in your routine.

TRACK YOUR PROGRESS

Another effective way to stay motivated is by tracking your progress. When you're in the middle of your fitness journey, it can be easy to overlook how far you've come. Keeping a workout journal or using a fitness app can help you see your improvements over time, whether it's in the number of reps you can do, the amount of time you can hold a plank, or even how you feel after a workout.

Celebrating small victories is crucial. Every time you hit a milestone, take a moment to acknowledge your hard work. This could be as simple as rewarding yourself with a new piece of workout gear or treating yourself to a relaxing day off. These rewards serve as positive reinforcement, helping to maintain your motivation as you continue to progress.

MIX IT UP

One of the quickest ways to lose motivation is to fall into a monotonous routine. Keep your workouts exciting by mixing things up. Try new exercises, change the order of your routine, or even take your workout outside for a change of scenery. The variety not only keeps you engaged but also challenges your muscles in new ways, preventing plateaus.

According to a study published in the Journal of Sport and Exercise Psychology, individuals who varied their exercise routine were 45% more likely to stick with their program compared to those who did the same workout every day.

ACCOUNTABILITY MATTERS

Having someone to keep you accountable can make all the difference. Whether it's a workout buddy, a coach, or even an online community, sharing your goals and progress with others can help you stay committed. Knowing that someone else is invested in your journey gives you that extra push to keep going, even on days when you're tempted to skip your workout.

OVERCOMING PLATEAUS: WHEN TO CHANGE YOUR ROUTINE

AS YOU PROGRESS IN YOUR CALISTHENICS JOURNEY, YOU MAY ENCOUNTER PLATEAUS—THOSE FRUSTRATING PERIODS WHEN YOUR PROGRESS SEEMS TO STALL, AND NO MATTER HOW HARD YOU WORK, YOU DON'T SEE THE SAME RESULTS. PLATEAUS ARE A NATURAL PART OF ANY FITNESS JOURNEY, BUT THEY CAN BE DISHEARTENING IF YOU'RE NOT PREPARED TO DEAL WITH THEM. UNDERSTANDING WHY PLATEAUS OCCUR AND KNOWING WHEN AND HOW TO CHANGE YOUR ROUTINE CAN HELP YOU PUSH THROUGH THESE CHALLENGING PHASES.

RECOGNIZING THE SIGNS OF A PLATEAU

The first step in overcoming a plateau is recognizing when you've hit one. Signs include a lack of progress in strength, endurance, or muscle growth, feeling bored or unchallenged by your workouts, or a general sense of fatigue and lack of motivation. If you notice any of these, it's time to evaluate your routine.

WHY PLATEAUS HAPPEN

Plateaus occur when your body becomes accustomed to your current workout regimen. Over time, your muscles adapt to the exercises you're doing, which means they no longer have to work as hard to perform the same movements. This adaptation is why you stop seeing progress.

Fitness expert Mark Verstegen explains, "Your body is incredibly efficient at adapting to stress.

If you're doing the same exercises over and over, your body will eventually become more efficient at those movements, leading to fewer gains. The key is to continually challenge your body in new ways."

HOW TO BREAK THROUGH A PLATEAU

To break through a plateau, you need to challenge your body with something new. This could mean increasing the intensity of your workouts, trying new exercises, or even changing the order in which you perform your exercises. For example, if you typically do push-ups at the start of your workout, try doing them at the end when your muscles are already fatigued.

Another strategy is to incorporate more advanced calisthenics movements into your routine. Moves like handstand push-ups, muscle-ups, or one-arm push-ups require greater strength and coordination, pushing your muscles to adapt and grow.

Research published in Medicine & Science in Sports & Exercise found that individuals who varied their resistance training exercises saw a 58% increase in muscle strength compared to those who did not vary their routines.

LISTEN TO YOUR BODY

While it's important to push through plateaus, it's equally important to listen to your body. Sometimes, a plateau can be a sign that you're overtraining and need to rest. Incorporating rest days and focusing on recovery—like stretching, foam rolling, or even light yoga—can help your body recharge and come back stronger.

ADAPTING CALISTHENICS FOR TRAVEL OR BUSY LIFESTYLES

LIFE DOESN'T ALWAYS FOLLOW A PREDICTABLE PATTERN. WORK TRIPS, VACATIONS, OR JUST A PARTICULARLY HECTIC WEEK CAN THROW OFF YOUR ROUTINE. THE GOOD NEWS IS THAT CALISTHENICS IS ONE OF THE MOST ADAPTABLE FORMS OF EXERCISE, MAKING IT EASY TO STAY CONSISTENT, NO MATTER WHERE YOU ARE OR HOW MUCH TIME YOU HAVE.

THE POWER OF BODYWEIGHT TRAINING

One of the best things about calisthenics is that you don't need any equipment. Your body is your gym. This makes it incredibly easy to do anywhere—whether you're in a hotel room, at a park, or even in your living room. A simple routine of push-ups, squats, planks, and lunges can give you a full-body workout without the need for any special equipment.

SHORT, HIGH-INTENSITY WORKOUTS

When time is tight, high-intensity interval training (HIIT) is your best friend. HIIT workouts involve short bursts of intense exercise followed by brief rest periods. These workouts can be done in as little as 15 to 20 minutes and are highly effective at burning fat and building strength. For example, you could do 30 seconds of push-ups, followed by 30 seconds of squats, then 30 seconds of planks, repeating the circuit three to four times.

PORTABLE EQUIPMENT FOR EXTRA CHALLENGE

While calisthenics is equipment-free, adding some portable tools can enhance your workouts. Resistance bands, for example, are lightweight and easy to pack. They can be used to add resistance to exercises like squats, lunges, and push-ups, making them more challenging. A suspension trainer, like TRX, is another great option that can be set up almost anywhere and provides a full-body workout using just your body weight.

STAYING ACTIVE ON THE GO

Beyond structured workouts, look for ways to stay active throughout your day, especially when traveling. Walk instead of taking a cab, use the stairs instead of the elevator, or do some stretching in your hotel room. Every little bit adds up, and these small efforts can help you maintain your fitness, even when you're away from your usual routine.

BUILDING A SUPPORT SYSTEM: COMMUNITY, ACCOUNTABILITY, AND PROGRESS SHARING

FITNESS IS NOT JUST A SOLO JOURNEY—IT'S A COMMUNITY EFFORT. SURROUNDING YOURSELF WITH LIKE-MINDED INDIVIDUALS CAN SIGNIFICANTLY BOOST YOUR MOTIVATION, KEEP YOU ACCOUNTABLE, AND MAKE THE ENTIRE PROCESS MORE ENJOYABLE. WHETHER IT'S AN ONLINE FORUM, A WORKOUT PARTNER, OR A LOCAL FITNESS GROUP, HAVING A SUPPORT SYSTEM CAN MAKE ALL THE DIFFERENCE.

THE IMPORTANCE OF ACCOUNTABILITY

Accountability is a powerful motivator. When you know that someone else is counting on you to show up, you're more likely to stick to your commitments. This is where workout partners or accountability buddies come into play. Find someone who shares similar fitness goals and check in with each other regularly. You can share your workout plans, update each other on your progress, and encourage one another on tough days.

ENGAGING WITH A COMMUNITY

Joining a fitness community, whether online or in person, provides a sense of belonging and support. These communities offer a platform to share your experiences, ask questions, and learn from others who are on the same journey. Online forums, social media groups, or even apps dedicated to calisthenics can connect you with people from around the world who share your passion.

SHARING YOUR PROGRESS

Sharing your progress, whether it's with your accountability partner or within a community, can be incredibly motivating. Documenting your journey through photos, videos, or even a fitness journal allows you to see how far you've come. It's easy to get caught up in the day-to-day and feel like you're not making progress, but looking back at where you started can be a powerful reminder of your achievements.

BUILDING LASTING RELATIONSHIPS

The relationships you build through your fitness journey can extend beyond just workouts. Many people find lifelong friends through their shared commitment to health and fitness. These connections can enrich your life, providing support not just in fitness but in other areas as well.

THE BOTTOM LINE

Fitness is a lifelong journey, not a quick fix. It's about making small, consistent efforts that add up over time. By creating a workout schedule that fits your life, staying motivated, overcoming plateaus, and adapting your routine to your lifestyle, you set yourself up for success. Remember, the goal is not to be perfect but to be consistent.

Surround yourself with a supportive community, stay accountable, and celebrate your progress along the way. Your efforts, no matter how small they may seem, are paving the way for a healthier, stronger, and more resilient you. Keep going—you've got this.

CONCLUSION

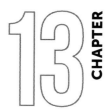

You've made it to the final chapter, and that's no small feat. Whether you've been diligently following each exercise or perhaps taking the journey at your own pace, you've invested time and energy into understanding the art of calisthenics. And as you stand at this point, it's crucial to realize that this isn't just the end of a book—it's the beginning of something much more significant.

FINAL THOUGHTS: THE LIFELONG BENEFITS OF CALISTHENICS

CALISTHENICS IS MORE THAN A WORKOUT ROUTINE; IT'S A PHILOSOPHY, A WAY OF LIFE THAT CAN SHAPE NOT JUST YOUR BODY BUT ALSO YOUR MIND AND SPIRIT. THE BENEFITS YOU'VE GAINED THROUGHOUT THIS JOURNEY ARE NOT FLEETING. THEY'RE THE FOUNDATIONS OF A LIFELONG PURSUIT OF FITNESS, WELLNESS, AND PERSONAL GROWTH. THE STRENGTH, FLEXIBILITY, AND MENTAL RESILIENCE YOU'VE BUILT THROUGH CALISTHENICS ARE TOOLS THAT WILL SERVE YOU WELL BEYOND THE CONFINES OF THIS BOOK.

THE PHYSICAL AND MENTAL TRANSFORMATIONS

When you first started, maybe you were looking to build muscle, lose weight, or just feel better in your own skin. And while those are all valid reasons to take up calisthenics, the true rewards of this practice go far deeper. The physical transformations are tangible—you can see and feel them with every push-up, pull-up, and squat. But what about the mental and emotional changes? Have you noticed how your confidence has grown with each challenge you've conquered? That's the power of calisthenics—it's a practice that not only sculpts your body but also sharpens your mind and fortifies your spirit.

According to research, regular physical activity, especially a practice as disciplined as calisthenics, has been shown to reduce symptoms of anxiety and depression, boost cognitive function, and improve overall mental well-being. This isn't just about getting stronger; it's about becoming the best version of yourself, inside and out.

THE JOY OF MASTERY

One of the greatest gifts calisthenics offers is the joy of mastery. Remember the first time you attempted a movement that seemed impossible? Maybe it was a muscle-up or a one-arm push-up. At first, it felt like a distant dream, something only elite athletes could achieve. But with time, practice, and perseverance, you did it. And that feeling—the rush of accomplishing something you once thought unattainable—is priceless.

This journey of mastery is ongoing. There will always be new skills to learn and new challenges to overcome. This is what makes calisthenics a lifelong pursuit. You're never done growing, improving, or learning. There's always another level to reach, another goal to set. And that's something to celebrate. Because in calisthenics, as in life, the journey is the reward.

HOW TO CONTINUE PROGRESSING BEYOND THE BOOK

NOW THAT YOU'VE BUILT A STRONG FOUNDATION, YOU MIGHT BE WONDERING, "WHAT'S NEXT?" THE BEAUTY OF CALISTHENICS IS THAT THERE'S ALWAYS ROOM FOR GROWTH AND ALWAYS A NEW CHALLENGE ON THE HORIZON. HOWEVER, TO KEEP PROGRESSING, YOU NEED TO APPROACH YOUR TRAINING WITH INTENTION AND ADAPTABILITY.

SETTING NEW GOALS

One of the most effective ways to continue progressing is by setting new goals. These goals should be specific, measurable, and aligned with your overall fitness aspirations. For instance, if you've mastered the basics, perhaps it's time to tackle more advanced movements like the front lever or the planche. These are not just physical goals—they're tests of your patience, persistence, and mental toughness.

When setting goals, remember to celebrate the small victories along the way. Each step forward, no matter how minor it may seem, is progress. And it's important to recognize and appreciate the effort you're putting in.

DIVERSIFYING YOUR TRAINING

While calisthenics offers a vast array of exercises and progressions, it's beneficial to diversify your training. This doesn't mean abandoning calisthenics but rather incorporating different styles and techniques to keep your routine fresh and engaging. For example, integrating elements of yoga can enhance your flexibility and mental focus, while high-intensity interval training (HIIT) can improve your cardiovascular endurance.

By diversifying your training, you not only prevent burnout but also ensure that you're developing a well-rounded physique. Each discipline complements the other, creating a holistic approach to fitness that addresses strength, flexibility, endurance, and mental resilience.

EMBRACING THE PLATEAU

Every athlete, regardless of experience level, hits a plateau at some point. It's that frustrating moment when progress seems to stall, no matter how hard you train. But here's the thing: a plateau isn't a sign of failure. It's an opportunity.

When you hit a plateau, it's a signal that your body has adapted to your current routine. This is when you need to mix things up—try new exercises, adjust your rep schemes, or experiment with different training intensities. Sometimes, the key to breaking through a plateau is as simple as giving your body the rest it needs to recover and grow.

And don't forget the mental aspect. Plateaus can be disheartening, but they're also a test of your resilience. Pushing through a plateau requires mental toughness and a deep belief in your ability to overcome obstacles. Embrace the challenge, and remember that progress isn't always linear. Sometimes, you need to take a step back to leap forward.

STAYING ENGAGED AND EVOLVING YOUR PRACTICE OVER TIME

AS YOU CONTINUE ON YOUR CALISTHENICS JOURNEY, IT'S IMPORTANT TO STAY ENGAGED AND KEEP EVOLVING YOUR PRACTICE. THIS IS WHERE MANY PEOPLE STRUGGLE—THEY START STRONG, BUT OVER TIME, MOTIVATION WANES, AND THEY LOSE THEIR DRIVE. SO HOW DO YOU KEEP THE FIRE BURNING?

BUILDING A COMMUNITY

One of the most powerful ways to stay motivated is by building or joining a community. Whether it's an online group, a local calisthenics class, or just a few friends who share your passion, being part of a community can provide support, inspiration, and accountability. When you train with others, you're more likely to push yourself harder, try new things, and stick with your routine. A community also offers a platform for learning and sharing. You can exchange tips, celebrate each other's successes, and help each other through challenges. It turns what can be a solitary pursuit into a shared journey filled with camaraderie and mutual growth.

CONTINUOUSLY LEARNING

Another key to staying engaged is adopting a mindset of continuous learning. Calisthenics is an ever-evolving field, with new techniques, exercises, and insights emerging all the time. Stay curious—read books, watch tutorials, attend workshops. The more you learn, the more you'll realize how much there is to discover. This continuous learning extends beyond just physical techniques. Dive into the science of training, nutrition, and recovery. Understanding the why behind what you do can deepen your appreciation for the practice and keep you motivated to keep improving.

REFLECTING ON YOUR JOURNEY

Finally, take time to reflect on how far you've come. It's easy to get caught up in the pursuit of the next goal, but it's equally important to look back and appreciate the progress you've made. Reflecting on your journey helps you stay grounded and reminds you of why you started in the first place. Journaling can be a great way to track your progress, both physically and mentally. Write down your goals, your challenges, and your triumphs. Over time, you'll have a record of your journey that you can look back on with pride.

ADAPTING TO LIFE'S CHANGES

Life is unpredictable, and your ability to adapt will determine the longevity of your calisthenics practice. There will be times when life gets in the way—whether it's due to work, family, or unexpected events. The key is to stay flexible in your approach. Even if you can't stick to your regular routine, find ways to keep moving, even if it's just a quick workout at home or a walk around the block.

Remember, calisthenics isn't just about achieving specific physical goals. It's about maintaining a lifestyle of movement, health, and well-being. As long as you keep that mindset, you'll find ways to stay active, no matter what life throws your way.

EMBRACING THE JOURNEY AHEAD

As you close this book, know that your journey with calisthenics is just beginning. The knowledge, skills, and mindset you've gained are tools that will serve you for a lifetime. You now have the foundation to continue growing, evolving, and pushing your limits.

Calisthenics is a journey of self-discovery and transformation. It's about more than just physical strength; it's about resilience, discipline, and the unending pursuit of bettering yourself. Whether you're aiming to master advanced movements, maintain your current level of fitness, or simply enjoy the process of moving your body, you're on a path that has no end.

So keep pushing. Keep exploring. And most importantly, keep enjoying the journey. Because in the end, it's not just about the destination—it's about the lifelong adventure of becoming the best version of yourself.

And remember, every time you step up to that pull-up bar, every time you drop down for a push-up, you're doing more than just working out. You're building a stronger, healthier, more resilient you. And that, above all, is what makes this journey worth every moment. The road ahead is full of potential. Now, it's up to you to seize it.

Made in the USA
Middletown, DE
09 February 2025

71045542R00095